Harmonic
Healing

Harmonic Healing

A Guide to Facilitated Oscillatory Release and Other Rhythmic Myofascial Techniques

Zachary Comeaux, DO, FAAO

Foreword by
Kenneth E. Nelson, DO, FAAO, FACOFP

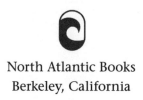

North Atlantic Books
Berkeley, California

Published by

North Atlantic Books
P.O. Box 12327
Berkeley, California 94712

Cover and book design by Jan Camp

Printed in the United States of America

Harmonic Healing: A Guide to Facilitated Oscillatory Release and Other Rhythmic Myofascial Techniques is sponsored by the Society for the Study of Native Arts and Sciences, a nonprofit educational corporation whose goals are to develop an educational and cross-cultural perspective linking various scientific, social, and artistic fields; to nurture a holistic view of arts, sciences, humanities, and healing; and to publish and distribute literature on the relationship of mind, body, and nature.

North Atlantic Books' publications are available through most bookstores. For further information, call 800-733-3000 or visit our website at www.northatlanticbooks.com.

Library of Congress Cataloging-in-Publication Data

Comeaux, Zachary.
Harmonic healing : facilitated oscillatory release and other rhythmic connective tissue techniques / Zachary Comeaux.
       p. ; cm.
Includes bibliographical references and index.
ISBN 978-1-55643-694-9 (alk. paper)
1. Manipulation (Therapeutics) 2. Oscillations--Therapeutic use. 3. Osteopathic medicine. 4. Connective tissues. I. Title.
[DNLM: 1. Manipulation, Osteopathic--methods. 2. Connective Tissue. WB 940 C732h 2008]
RZ342.C66 2008
615.8'2—dc22
200800317

1 2 3 4 5 6 7 8 9 UNITED GRAPHICS 14 13 12 11 10 09 08

This work is dedicated to my mother, Mary, who taught me to value reading and writing, and my father, Zachary Sr., who taught me to plan and to work with my hands.

Contents

Part II: Principles and Support for Facilitated Oscillatory Release 77

Illustrations

Foreword

This text represents a landmark contribution to the literature of bodywork, in general, and to that of osteopathy, in particular. It describes how manipulative procedures may be applied from a physiological perspective, as well as from an anatomical perspective.

As every osteopathic student knows, osteopathy began as a thorough understanding of the machinery of life in the mind and nurturing hands of Andrew Taylor Still. The Old Doctor is known to have said that anatomy, anatomy, and anatomy are the three most important subjects that any student of osteopathy must come to know. But, for any machine to function, to be alive in this case, there must be motivating force. Still understood this. He recognized that there must be a *life force*. In the light of his intense faith, and because of the limitations of medical science in the nineteenth century, he succinctly explained that vital force as the action of the Divine Creator.

John Martin Littlejohn, one of Still's early students, and an osteopathic visionary, realized that human physiology provided the key to understanding the machinery of life's motivating force. In an article published in 1902 in the *Journal of the American Osteopathic Association,* entitled "The Physiological Basis of the Therapeutic Law," Littlejohn stated: "All life represents forces and the nature of this force is rhythmic or vibratile, because the disorder is maladjustment, the two possible conditions being above or below par or normal, and vibratility or motility can only be changed by something of its own nature." Thus Littlejohn was considering somatic dysfunction and the focus of manipulative treatment in the context of rhythmic physiology, i.e., the life force, and not just in the anatomical, mechanical, context. This difference in perspective contributed to the parting of ways between Still and Littlejohn, with their influences ultimately manifesting on opposite sides of the Atlantic Ocean.

This is not to say that the American osteopathic tradition has not taken the physiological impact of somatic dysfunction into consideration. The work of such brilliant researchers as Louisa Burns, Korr and Denslow, and others has diligently sought out the physiology of somatic dysfunction, i.e., affect. But somatic dysfunction has, by the majority of practitioners, always been viewed in a mechanical rather than a physiological context.

In this text Zachary Comeaux has reunited the physiological and mechanical in a complete view of dysfunction as, not only, a restriction of motion, but also as a dysrhythmia. He goes on to consider the therapeutic impact of controlled oscillation imparted by the practitioner upon the patient and the effect that should have upon somatic dysfunction by the reestablishment of normal physiological rhythm.

Most all practitioners of manual therapeutics are aware of the significance placed upon oscillatory rhythms in some aspects of osteopathic theory and practice. Certainly the 0.10- to 0.15-Hz frequency oscillation of the cranial rhythmic impulse (CRI) of W. G. Sutherland's osteopathy in the cranial field comes immediately to mind. In this paradigm, the incitant procedure of temporal rocking or the focused application of the CRI in V-spread are both examples of therapeutically controlled oscillation. The percussion hammer of Robert Fulford is another such example. But there are many more examples that we may not right away consider. Among the first therapeutic procedures taught to osteopathic students is the soft-tissue stretching of the spinal paravertebral musculature. The student is taught to laterally stretch the paravertebral soft tissues, to gently release them, and then to repeat the process. The aware student quickly realizes that there is a comfortable rate with which this procedure can be applied. One may have had a similar experience when performing rib raising or the pedal fascial lymphatic pump of Dalrymple. As Dr. Comeaux points out, the body will respond optimally when therapeutic manual procedures are applied rhythmically and at the proper frequency. Not just in the case of the examples here listed, but for essentially all types of manipulative treatment from cranial and indirect functional to direct articulatory and even high-velocity low-amplitude procedures. Additionally, Dr. Comeaux shows us that the application of vibratory forces may be employed diagnostically like sonar, and in skilled hands can pinpoint a locus of dysfunctional restriction.

The text is very readably organized, with enough history to allow the reader to follow the development of thought regarding therapeutic vibration over the past century in North America and Europe. It provides a well-referenced description of bioenergetics and the neurophysiology supporting physiological oscillation from the subcellular level to the tensegrity model of Donald Ingber. Dr. Comeaux then describes his own contribution, Facilitated Oscillatory Release, and provides the reader with well-written descriptions of its diagnostic methods and therapeutic procedures. The text is completed with a good number of treatment examples to provide the reader with an understanding of practical application.

This book is not a reductionist, single-procedure type of presentation. It is not a description of one more brand of manual treatment to be added to the already overburdened pantheon of named subsets of manipulation. It is, rather, an all-embracing addition to everyone's diagnostic and therapeutic armamentarium. More important, it allows us to look at somatic dysfunction in the context of physiology as John Martin Littlejohn envisioned it more than a century ago, and in doing so it bridges the Atlantic Ocean, reuniting the osteopaths of many countries and continents.

I can honestly say that this little tome is well worth the time you will invest in reading, and rereading, it.

Kenneth E. Nelson, DO, FAAO, FACOFP

September 22, 2007

Lyon, France

Acknowledgments

Special thanks for help or influence in the process of developing this book rightfully go to colleagues who have listened, traded ideas, or afforded me the opportunity to publish the emerging thoughts in journal format. Among these are Robert Fulford, Anthony Chila, John Howell, Jean Guy Sicotte, Leon Chaitow, Christian Fossum, John Wernham, Laurie Hartman, and the Committee on Fellowship of the American Academy of Osteopathy.

Credit goes to Karen Steele, David Essig-Beatty, and Bill Lemley for affording me the opportunity to introduce these ideas into the undergraduate curriculum at the West Virginia School of Osteopathic Medicine, and the students and patients who have inadvertently served as a learning laboratory for my evolving technique.

Thanks go also to Eric Miller and Trista Bowles for assisting with the photography.

Loving thanks go to my wife Linda, who provides a base of support from which it is possible to write cogent ideas. As I revise this manuscript, in view of snow-capped Colorado peaks, she tempts me to be playing with the grandchildren.

Introduction

Connective Tissues, Bioenergetics, and Rhythm

Overview

Rhythmic activity and periodic motion are fundamental aspects of all life function. The beat of our heart, the daily sun cycle, and the cricket on a summer's night remind us of this. But this theme is repeated in molecular and cellular processes and tissue organization, as well as posture and locomotion. Consequently, rhythmicity has a natural place in those therapeutic disciplines that intend to restore health by restoring natural motion to the body. This book introduces, or renews an appreciation for, the value of rhythmic motion in diagnosis and treatment in bodywork. It intends to be fun, scholarly yet practical.

The field of manual therapies is broad and diverse. A number of bodywork methods, including osteopathy, have used oscillatory maneuvers, but only marginally. We will review this history and then look at the contemporary use of rhythmic motion in bodywork with special focus on osteopathic approaches. Following this we will introduce and describe an organized, practical approach to integrating the use of oscillatory force, under the title Facilitated Oscillatory Release (FOR). To make this method useful to a wider community of bodywork practitioners, we will compare FOR to other rhythmic manual modalities. Since I intend to introduce FOR as an extension of connective tissue or myofascial release techniques in general usage, the theoretical basis of these models, and their extension in adding oscillation, are reviewed in these pages.

Despite the fact that I teach and practice as an osteopathic physician, it is my contention that the methods described may be applied in a broader bodywork context.

FOR is intended to suggest principles of application, not to present a series of exercises to be imitated routinely. It integrates well into a variety of current models of manual treatment in body culture. And for those less familiar and desiring a further appreciation of the osteopathic context in which FOR was developed, Appendix A describes the osteopathic approach to manual therapy in more detail.

For those interested in an energy medicine approach but feeling out of synchrony with scientific physiology, as well as those with an interest in physiology who feel estranged from advocates of energy medicine, this book is intended to provide a bridge. The material contained here, frequently taught as part of a course entitled Bioenergetically Integrated Osteopathic Medicine, represents an inclusive synthesis, rather than a new field of study. As a result, although growing from an aspect of osteopathy, the principles and background of FOR are easily adapted to physical therapy, physical medicine and rehabilitation, or other bodywork disciplines.

Despite interdisciplinary differences, historically osteopathic thought has been a watershed for other bodyworkers. Principles of counterstrain, myofascial release, muscle energy, and craniosacral work, pioneered by osteopaths, have found resonance, if not adaptation, in a variety of manual approaches. Since the beginning of osteopathy, when Andrew Taylor Still cited the importance of the fascias of the body, practitioners have been methodically approaching the connective tissue matrix as a key to healing. In putting connective tissue work in context, Still writes:

> I write at length of the universality of the fascia to impress the reader with the idea that this connecting substance must be free at all parts to receive and discharge all fluids, and to appropriate and use them in sustaining animal life, and eject all impurities, that health may not be impaired by dead and poisonous fluids. A knowledge of the universal extent of the fascias is imperative, and is one of the greatest aids to the person who seeks the causes of disease. The fascia and its nerves demand his attention, and on his knowledge of them much of his success depends.[1]

Again:

The fascia proves itself to be the matrix of life and death.[2]

This thread of manual work has been variously named and described under the headings of Connective Tissue Release,[3] Myofascial Release,[4] Ligamentous Articular Release,[5] Still Technique,[6] and Balanced Ligamentous Tension.[7] A common feature of these methods is the continual use of feedback for diagnostic purposes during a dialogic encounter with the body's connective tissues. However, each expression of these methods, whether articular or regional in its focus, tends to begin with the practitioner approaching and engaging the patient in a static resting posture. Active motion testing, passive linear stretch, tension reduction, or articular circumduction are then induced to test and alter tissue characteristics.

For the most part, passivity on the part of the patient is assumed; it is considered essential in assessing tissue resting tone, a baseline for assessing isolated active motion, and helpful in inducing release through relaxation when appropriate. In the largely passive state, the quality and quantity of native motion are often deduced rather than observed. Admittedly, there is at times a more complex interaction between practitioner and patient in guiding progressive active motion testing. But this range of motion testing can give only one dimension of native motion characteristics. It still does not replicate the rhythmicity of routine bodily activity, such as gait. Could palpation occur in a patient in a more dynamic state?

Although we teach observation of gait, it is impractical, while observing, to palpate and treat the walking patient. However, I and others in contemporary and historic times have intuitively used rhythmic movement in the course of work with connective tissue. Nevertheless, this aspect of working has received limited verbal expression overall in the field of manual work, including osteopathy. Dr. Still frequently reflected on being directed in manual treatment by discovery of the abnormal structure or function and returning that aspect of the patient to its normal relationship. Despite our habit of concentrating on the description of the body in static dysfunctional states, or at the beginning or end range of motion, the body is inherently rhythmic in function. Gait, respiration, and cardiac rhythm are commonly recognized as reflecting this reality. Yet in most diagnostic and treatment contexts, the appreciation of the deeper physiological significance of rhythmicity and the use of rhythmic motion have not been so frequently described.

This book is intended to highlight and support the work of those who have felt an urge to incorporate rhythmic movement during diagnosis and treatment. It begins with a discussion of the utility of the connective tissue approach to the body in manual therapy. Then it will further develop an appreciation for the potential effects of rhythmic force on this connective tissue system as well as exploring the inherent rhythmic function of specialized connective tissue, namely, the neuromuscular system.

Besides being effective, performing good manipulative treatment should be fun. Part of the fun is continual discovery, learning more about the human condition, and expanding our individual skills. Hopefully, this book will also help to support this process.

Part I documents the history of the use of rhythmic oscillation in motion testing and treatment. Attention is given to those who have attempted, based on their experience, to systematize an approach to the integration of oscillation in bodywork. This has occurred on both sides of the Atlantic and within and outside of work that is primarily osteopathic.

Part II expands both the rationale and the application of the use of oscillatory force in a clinical context. It draws on a diverse selection of contemporary neurophysiological research describing the intricate functional patterns of rhythmic coordination involved in postural and voluntary motion in the body. This synthesis of neurophysiology is presented to provide credibility for the use of rhythmic motion in therapeutics. However, scientific proofs are limited because of the ethics involved in human experimentation and in the limitations of parallelism in nonhuman animal research. Most patients complain of pain presenting at a lower level of threat to survival than is involved in most nonhuman animal experimental models. Also, the subjective aspects of pain interact with emotional aspects of the human psyche (fear, guilt, revenge, depression), none of which are reliably communicated by our animal research subjects. Despite these limitations, a significant body of contemporary physiological research supports the relevance of oscillatory rhythms in the body's coordinative functions. However, our presentation remains a model. And so, in this context, we can add *coordinative dysrhythmia* to the list of effects of trauma or strain reflected in the patient's symptoms. Correspondingly, we can add the return of harmonic rhythmic function as a goal of manipulative treatment. This is the main theme developed in this text.

Practical applications of these considerations in my clinical experience have been formulated under the descriptive term of Facilitated Oscillatory Release (FOR). The association of these ideas and tactics as a rhythmic extension of connective tissue release will become clear.

I have selected the term Facilitated Oscillatory Release as a descriptor in the initial writing on this theme. FOR is not intended as a separate method. It represents an attempt to systematize a number of empirically derived and effective applications of rhythmic movement consistent with scientific modeling and hypothetical mechanisms that describe the effectiveness. The method draws heavily on the historical research material summarized in this book, but has many distinctive features. FOR, since it is not a stand-alone method, integrates well into the other methods commonly used in osteopathic clinical practice and other physical disciplines. Most particularly, it is seen as an extension of connective tissue release as taught by Anthony Chila, DO. However, since our first meetings, both of us have reformulated our thought in light of the work of the late Robert Fulford, DO, who personally touched our lives. Dr. Fulford's use of the percussion vibrator to instill therapeutic oscillation helped stimulate my interest in the oscillatory dimension of manual work.

For those with primary interest in FOR, please begin reading in Chapters 8, 9, and 10.

Connective Tissue Methods

For the sake of clarity as we proceed, it is my intent to use the descriptors *connective tissue* and *myofascial,* despite legitimate differences in application, as equivalent terms in this text.

Connective tissue techniques rely on various methods of returning the tissue to a state of normal balance of tensions that existed prior to a reaction to trauma or strain. In doing so, it is hoped that there is a return to normal body function and the disappearance of pain or other symptoms. Working effectively with this balance relies on an understanding of the qualities and properties of the tissue engaged, many of which are determined by its chemical structure. The biochemical nature of the tissue determines its native properties as well as its response to strain. Routine distention of tissue in its elastic range is largely due to alterations in the amorphous matrix or ground substance. Such reversible deformational change (creep) will usually return to more normal, resting length since the potential bond energy is conserved in the tissue in readily accessible state.[8] Sometimes it needs help from a perceptive practitioner, to redistribute forces; this is one basis for therapy. However, recurrent strain, as in overuse syndrome, may result in fibrin buildup to reinforce native tissue where increased demand requires increased strength to limit further injury. This stiffening of tissue may strongly affect the function of other tissue due to spatial crowding or loss of native flexibility.

Additionally, the natural healing process that results in fibrin production may limit some aspect of joint, vascular, or nerve function. A focal example of this is persistent inflammation (a natural healing activity) associated with the articular capsule or the synovial lining of a joint. Although the physiological intent is joint protection, exaggerated healing may limit proper function, resulting in restriction of motion or pain.

Furthermore, if connective tissue experiences a still higher degree of force, plastic deformation may occur in which the fibrin matrix undergoes a disconnect-reconnect event between individual molecules while the gross tissue remains intact. Because this process involves the dissipation of mechanical energy (hysteresis), tissue does not naturally return to its initial resting length with the release of strain.[9]

These stages are potentially progressive for each individual fiber in the tissue. When cumulative distention of sufficient fibers occurs beyond the point of maximal plastic deformation, repair is more complex. Native healing may result in fibrin scarring through granulation, but may be facilitated by surgical repair. If native repair results in joint hypermobility and instability, prolotherapy may be helpful.

Embriologically, muscle tissue is derived from the same mesodermal tissue as fascial connective tissue.[10] Additionally, it possesses the capacity to resist strain or create voluntary motion through contraction or shortening of individual fibers. This function enables the body to resist the force of gravity to engage in stance and alter stance to create locomotion. Often the innervation and proprioceptive regulation of striated muscle tissue would seem to differentiate it from fascia or other identifiable muscle tissue. However, contractile elements have been identified in fascia. This being so, the commonalities between classic myofascial work and muscle-related techniques become more numerous. Regardless, connective tissue completely invests muscle fibers and the gross structure of muscle. Although the topic of normalization of muscle tone in manual work is a very broad one, beyond the scope of this book, I wish to make a bridge of relevance between connective tissue or myofascial release techniques, and the various techniques that focus on normalization of muscle tone (counterstrain, muscle energy technique, and so on). It is my contention that because of the intimate relationships in structure and function of muscle and fibrous connective tissue, many of the same operational physiological principles apply to both fields of endeavor. This will have relevance when we look in Chapter 8 at the physiological basis for the technique described as Facilitated Oscillatory Release.

The characteristics of specific connective tissues vary according to their particular location in the complex organization of the body and their resultant function. When trauma inhibits this function, the application of connective tissue techniques varies according to the symptoms and the structural and functional characteristics, including the configuration of the tissues affected. This is the underlying theme—that FOR, and oscillatory force in general, should be applied according to the practitioner's theoretical basis, knowledge, intent, and license. It is not an isolated system of manual practice, nor a separate osteopathic model.

As mentioned above, the connective tissue approach to healing tissue injury has developed into a variety of methods, each with a slightly different emphasis on details of diagnosis and treatment. Some authors describe the application of a sustained linear stretch as the activating corrective force. My introduction to connective tissue technique followed the line of thought from Still, Sutherland, Becker (Rollin), and Chila, and has included this principle. Coupled with this approach is the so-called indirect myofascial technique, which intends to facilitate the return of tissue to native state after sustained creep phenomenon in another way. This method listens and follows the tissues' preference for reorganization and cooperates in creating conditions for the gentle facilitated further expression of these preferences. Spontaneous reorganization often occurs. However, it may be obstructed by the emotional memory of traumatic events. The practitioner may elect also to address this level of tissue distortion. In any case, the practitioner's role is as a catalyst in the process rather than as the one directing it.

Admittedly, indirect methods of connective tissue release are less invasive, involving gentle compression of the target tissue to allow for fibrin and collagen reorganization within the medium of the ground substance. However, in practice, the method often begins with the discrete application of an initiating force before following the body's preferred pattern of reorganization.[11]

In addition to these two approaches, direct and indirect connective tissue release, there has also been a long-standing tendency by intuitive practitioners to use repetitive corrective force or oscillatory motion in the application of ligamentous articular or fascial stretch.[12] Still's famous resting of his neck on a rope swing seems to include the potential for rhythmic repetitive stretch.[13] As we will see below, there have been several attempts to integrate oscillation formally into manipulative protocols. Still's early students, including John Martin Littlejohn, picked up on this theme from their mentor.

Rhythmic motion may effect change by applying small incremental stretches, induce the reversal of creep sustained in injury, or replenish energy lost through hysteresis. The neuroreflexive entrainment possible with oscillation is dealt with in depth in Chapter 8.

Fulford's Approach to Vibrational Manipulation

As mentioned, I was introduced to the clinical application of oscillatory force by Robert Fulford's use of the percussion vibrator or "hammer" in the context of osteopathic manipulation.[14,15] Some suggest that the methods and principles described by Fulford are eccentric to the main body of osteopathic work. His attention to what he called the "ethric body" or human energy field leads some practitioners to be distracted from the valuable features of Fulford's work, which are compatible with and complementary to the progression of traditional osteopathic thought. Fulford's approach is discussed in Chapter 5, but for those interested in more detail, it can also be found in the works cited in the references for this Introduction.

Impressed by the effectiveness of Fulford's method, I have worked in two directions. One has been to increase credibility for this model by exploring current physiological research data that would further elucidate the mechanisms and relationships that underlie its effectiveness. The second direction had been to develop or refine, in a systematic way, a manual application of similar methods and principles, more compatible with and integrated into other contemporary osteopathic treatment models. This effort has resulted in the teaching and publication of the principles and protocols called Facilitated Oscillated Release.

Relevance to Other Manual and Osteopathic Work

In the process of this development, however, I have become aware of the work of other individuals who have included rhythmic or oscillatory methods as a main or significant mode of working. Trager work, Harmonic Release, and Torque Unwinding are some examples. Also, the field of physical therapy has integrated, under the themes of peripheral neural facilitation and post-isometric release, principles compatible with this current work. Geographic, cultural, and political distances have impeded communication and recognition of the similarities and differences between these approaches. This text is an effort to bring together a summary of developed models that build on the body's functional rhythmicity and a collection of physiological research that underpins these practices. Additionally, the rhythmic neural coordinative phenomena cited may well be useful in understanding the alteration in tissue texture and hypertonic muscle associated with musculoskeletal dysfunction more broadly.

References

[1] Still, Andrew. *Philosophy and Mechanical Principles of Osteopathy* (Kirksville, Mo.: Osteopathic Enterprises, 1986), 61. Originally published in 1892.

[2] Still, Andrew. *Philosophy of Osteopathy* (Indianapolis: American Academy of Osteopathy, 1977), 89. Originally self-published in Kirksville, Mo. in 1899.

[3] Chila, Anthony. "Ligamentous Articular Release," in Ward, Robert, ed. *Foundations for Osteopathic Medicine,* 2nd ed. (Philadelphia: Lippincott Williams and Wilkins, 2003), 908.

[4] Ward, Robert, ed. *Foundations for Osteopathic Medicine,* 2nd ed. (Philadelphia: Lippincott Williams and Wilkins, 2003), 931.

[5] Speece, Conrad A., and William Thomas Crow. *Ligamentous Articular Strain: Osteopathic Manipulative Techniques for the Body* (Seattle: Eastland Press, 2001).

[6] Van Buskirk, Richard. *Applications of a Rediscovered Technique of Andrew Taylor Still* (Indianapolis: American Academy of Osteopathic Medicine, 1999).

[7] Ward, Robert. Op. cit., 916.

[8] Lederman, E. *Fundamentals of Manual Therapy: Physiology, Neurology and Psychology* (New York: Churchill Livingston, 1997), 28.

[9] Adams, M., and Nicholai Bogduk. *The Biomechanics of Back Pain* (Edinburgh: Churchill Livingston 2002), 7.

[10] Moore, Keith, and T. Persaud. *The Developing Human,* 6th ed. (Philadelphia: W. B. Saunders, 1996), 87.

[11] Essig-Beatty, David. *Pocket Manual of OMT* (Lewisburg: West Virginia School of Osteopathic Medicine, 2004).

[12] Wernham, John. *Applied Osteopathic Therapeutics* (Maidstone, England: Institute of Classical Osteopathy, 1996).

[13] Still, Andrew. *Autobiography of A. T. Still* (Indianapolis: American Academy of Osteopathy, 1981), 32. Originally published in Colorado Springs, Colo., in 1908.

[14] Fulford, Robert. *Dr. Fulford's Touch of Life* (New York: Simon & Schuster, 1996).

[15] Comeaux, Zachary. *Robert Fulford, DO, and the Philosopher Physician* (Seattle: Eastland Press, 2002).

Part I

Conceptual Background for Oscillatory Manipulation

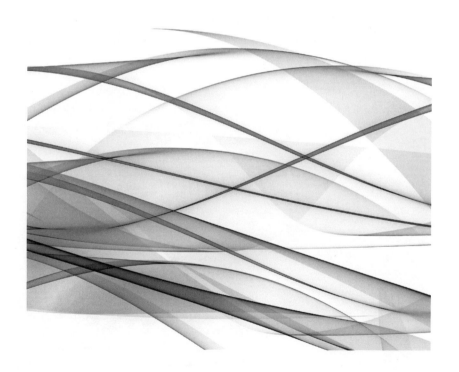

Chapter 1

Scope of the Work

The Issue of Scientific Credibility

In approaching the topic of rhythmic or vibratory motion in physical medicine, one has a decision to make regarding the scope of inquiry. Each of us experiences, or does not experience, the sense of relevance of various phenomena along the continuum of frequencies of repetitive motion or vibration. Although physics recognizes the concept of the electromagnetic spectrum, and the fact that some parts of the frequency range are sensible to all or most of us through particular sense modalities, there is no consensus about the relevance and significance of some portions of this spectrum of human experience to manual diagnosis and treatment. And so, the relevance of energy medicine is variable and slowly progressing. Some of this may change with increasing appreciation for the relevance of quantum physics and other more advanced concepts in physics to the field of bioscience. But this appreciation, though part of an active academic debate in the further understanding of human genomics, is in its infancy in the popular mind as well as that of the health care community.

In the process of biological discovery, what to some is considered scientific, conforming to a set standard of perception, measurability, and reproducibility, does not meet with the same interpretation by others. Occasionally, the means of observation may represent a specialty approach. Or conditions for reproducibility may prove difficult. Or again, the phenomenon may be known in a way that is not commonly accepted as observation.

In the context of these competing or complementary paradigms, I have tried in this book to keep within the scope of science as defined by the position based on empirical reproducibility, in order to make this work more universally usable. However, in clinical practice, as individuals are dealt with in their totality (or, as Still would say, as God created them), it is common to encounter and interact daily through more subtle channels with more subtle information. Most practitioners should feel comfortable wisely and sensitively incorporating all their talents into their work, including intuition, good will, and empathy. They understand that biomechanics, biodynamics, and bioenergetics are but complementary analytical perspectives of living systems.

Historically, there has been a truism that structure and function are interrelated. Yet, often this interrelationship has been interpreted to mean there is only one perspective from which to view the body and a "right" approach to diagnosis and treatment. Some argue that structure determines function; others that function molds structure. The consequence of this argument has often been a reductionistic approach. As a result of such selectivity, the role of certain other aspects of body function, including the fuller significance of rhythmic processes, have not been given full scientific credence but have been marginally expressed as vibrational medicine. The implication has been that they are esoteric and worthy only of anthropological or poetic interest, not true scientific study.

In Chapter 3 some of the historic attempts to blend the apparently contradictory aspects of empirical and intuitive reality in the definition of the person, our patient, are discussed.

Chapters 4, 5, and 6 document, compare, and contrast contemporary methods, both in Europe and America, that integrate oscillation or vibration as a crucial part of their methodologies.

Body Definition and Bioenergetics

The field of bioenergetics often remains a controversial topic despite the convergence of the fields of energetics and physics at the subatomic level,[1,2,3] and the application of these relationships in medical nuclear imaging, acupuncture, and MRI. The topic of bioenergetics, and the frontier between materialist reductionism and an expanded view of biology, has significant relevance to this present area of work and is reviewed briefly in Chapter 7. A discussion of some of these issues is also dealt with briefly in Chapter 4 in the section on Dr. Fulford's work.

However, despite the intuition of many astute clinicians, and isolated experimental work, the scientific explanation for the method of action or relationship of subtle bioenergetic phenomena remains to be well elucidated and accepted. As a result, explanations sometimes rely heavily on intercultural anthropological expressions, including religious symbolism and esoteric literature. The intent of this book is to wed clinical experience with a scientific support base. As a result, although we touch on it here, a full discussion of subtle electromagnetic and bioenergetics, which reflect a valid but different analytical perspective of living systems, will be reserved hopefully for a future book.

Chapter 8 provides a strong scientific foundation underpinning the rational use of rhythmic motion in communicating with and rebalancing a proprioceptive system that has accommodated serious stress. Chapter 9 describes the particular background, principles, and application exercises proper to FOR. Practical examples of clinical integration of FOR in patient management are shared in Chapter 10.

References

[1] Gerber, Richard. *Vibrational Medicine: New Choices for Healing Ourselves* (Santa Fe, N.M.: Bear and Co., 1988).

[2] Handoll, Nicholas. *Anatomy of Potency* (Hereford, England: Osteopathic Supply Ltd, 2000).

[3] Oschman, James. *Energy Medicine: The Scientific Basis* (Edinburgh, Scotland: Churchill Livingston, 2000).

Chapter 2

Active Connective Tissue—A Perspective

The Importance of Fascia

Generally speaking, in connective tissue work the influence of structure on function is critical at a fundamental level. Dr. Still expressed the importance of the fascia as the support for neural and vascular structures but more importantly as the medium of exchange of nutrients and immune factors, to the extent they were understood in his day.

For Still, the analysis of the structure and function of the body included assessment proceeding from the gross scale down to the cellular level, with reciprocal interaction between levels. In many places he appears to have insight into and describes what appears to be the cellular milieu. Although limited by the instrumentation of his day, he refers periodically to the atom as the fundamental constitutive particle of biological matter. Proper structural organization, on all levels, was important.

In Still's treatise on the comprehensive osteopathic approach to treating disease, *Osteopathy Research and Practice,* the Old Doctor makes this connection clear. In writing on the nutritive power of the nervous system, a key concept, he writes:

We find a nerve fiber, trace it to some locality and there we find a great number of capillary arteries in full action surrounding a nerve plexus with many branches coming to and going from it. Do these nerves absorb this blood and prepare it to be sent on to be applied in forming muscle and tissue? Let us reason cautiously because if the finale of the atoms of flesh is completed by the nerve system then we see that the two systems, nerve and blood supply, must be kept fully normal or we will fail to cure our patients. Let us remember that no atom of flesh in the body is out of connection with the three nerves, motor, nutritive and sensory, and that we should know that all muscles and other parts of the body are formed by and act through their nerve energy. In order to succeed in our profession we must work to establish and maintain normal nerved functioning and that can be done by adjusting all parts that would hinder in the least any perfect action of the three classes of nerves above named.[1]

It is easy to appreciate that although he was not educated in cellular metabolism, Still's "atoms of flesh" represent the same reality that we now describe as cells. For a complete appreciation of Still's physiology, it is helpful to couple this quote with the following one regarding the fascia from the *Philosophy and Mechanical Principles of Osteopathy:*

It [fascia] surrounds every muscle, vein and all organs of the body. It has a network of nerves, cells and tubes running to and from it: it is crossed and no doubt filled with millions of nerve centers and fibers which carry on the work of secreting and excreting fluids vital and destructive. By its actions we live and by its failures we die.

I write at length of the universality of the fascia to impress the reader with the idea that this connecting substance must be free at all parts to receive and discharge all fluids, and to appropriate and use them in sustaining animal life, and eject all impurities, that health may not be impaired by dead and poisonous fluids.[2]

The integrity of the structural elements was not an end in itself. Rather, structural integrity is key to the complementary function of vessels and nerves in health. Much of Still's thought here is encapsulated in the "principle" of the interrelationship of structure and function. However, somehow Still's interest in the fascia and its functional significance became largely drowned in the minds of his followers by one of his competing analogies, that of biomechanical organization of the joints or articulations of the skeletal system, as a machine.

Diverse Approaches to Working with Fascia

As we will see more fully in Chapter 4, one of Still's students, T.J. Ruddy, initiated a systematic way of cyclically activating this nerve/vascular/muscle conglomerate to overcome stasis, or suspension of function, Ruddy's and Still's descriptors for somatic dysfunction. The Facilitated Oscillatory Release methodology presented later in this book is to be viewed as a means to engage this same physiological functional loop, using externally induced passive motion to entrain and accelerate this system through rhythmic afferent stimulation.[3] Ruddy's work, as that of most others noted here briefly, will be further described later.

William Sutherland, a participant in Still's third graduating class, was inspired to focus on the theme of subtle function and subtle motion within the structure of the body, prompted by aspects of rhythmic respiratory motion. Based on his observations, initially in the head, or cranial region, his attention included the importance of the membranous or connective tissue structures in that area. He later expanded this emphasis to include ligamentous structures adjacent to the joints, which corresponded in function to the membranes of the cranium. The fascias were recognized as an extension of this connective tissue system in the periphery.[4]

Rollin Becker, one of Sutherland's students, practiced, taught, and wrote about a means of relating to and treating the fascial system from a phenomenological standpoint. An important aspect of his descriptions is the recognition that this system is alive, sensitive, expressive, and capable of dialogic communication with an alert and properly disposed practitioner.

Additionally, treatment of this system could be conducted as a dialogue with this coordinative system. Becker would express this as listening, and as taking the tissues where they expressed a preference to go.[5]

Becker's interpretation of his mentor's thought has evolved under the titles fascial ligamentous release technique and myofascial release as elaborations of this work.[6,7]

The work of Robert Fulford, also a student of Sutherland, emphasizes the bioelectrical subset of myofascial function. We will look at this work more at length in Chapter 4. However, in scope, each of these latter approaches represents a reductionism or extension of the conceptualization of the ligamentous and membranous system of Still and Sutherland.[8]

Mindful of the intent of Sutherland and Becker to describe the dynamic interrelationship reflected in the fascial system of the body as a total body operative principle, Anthony Chila, DO, has described this work as the connective tissue model. In this context, the permeating presence of connective tissue in bone, ligament, fascia, muscle, and nerve presents a point of engagement for both diagnosis and treatment. It is represented in personal communication as all-investing, as the "big bandage of the body." Although he must use structured protocols as teaching exercises, Chila actually teaches principles for engaging this living tissue system. Clinical application is rarely standardized. Rather, building on Becker, Chila engages individual local tissue elements or regionally associated functionally related structures in the treatment process, most often guided by the patient's nonverbal expression of need. The practitioner provides supportive guidance and gentle suggestion, intended to trace the tissue memory of trauma. This may facilitate spontaneous unwinding in linear, spiral, or diagonal graceful, sometime rhythmic, motion patterns. It is a dance. The practitioner provides continuous contact and support until release is achieved, integrating principles of direct and indirect applications of force. Respiratory cooperation is recruited as well as an intrinsic force to drive change. So too is the cranial rhythmic impulse used a parameter of diagnosis and prognosis.

The practitioner's interpretation of the body's intended motion includes appreciation of the organization and characteristics of the myofascial system. The patient's unwinding sequence relates very much to the difference between the native and traumatically altered disposition of this fascial envelope.

Sadly, this didactic material is available mostly through unpublished course notes from years of teaching. A brief synopsis is accessible in Ward's *Foundations for Osteopathic Medicine*.[9] Further material is available as taped or transcribed presentations at convocations of the American Academy of Osteopathy, especially in course notes from elective workshops given in 2003 and 2004.[10,11]

The perspective of Pierre Tricot, DO, smoothly integrates the idea of connective tissue, as all tissue, as having the distinct qualities of being alive and communicative, features often clinically overlooked. Although the theme of vibration or oscillation is not a major emphasis in this work, the message is clear that the nature of the person, and of individual tissues comprising the person, are more vital and dynamic than usually conceptualized. This helps support a transition to the use of rhythmic motion. He does so by emphasizing the engagement of cranial and peripheral tissue in a dynamic dialogical fashion. This broadens one's horizons and encourages us to reevaluate our understanding of the body, of the person.[12]

References

[1] Still, Andrew. *Osteopathy: Research and Practice* (Seattle: Eastland Press, 1992), 187. Originally self-published in Kirksville, Mo. in 1910.

[2] Still, Andrew. *Philosophy and Mechanical Principles of Osteopathy* (Kirksville, Mo.: Osteopathic Enterprises, 1986, originally published in 1892), 60, 61.

[3] Ruddy, T. J. "Osteopathic Rhythmic Resistive Duction Therapy," *Yearbook* (Academy of Applied Osteopathy, 1961), 58–68.

[4] Sutherland, William. *Teachings in the Science of Osteopathy,* Anne Wales, ed. (Dallas: Sutherland Cranial Teaching Foundation, 1990), 234.

[5] Becker, Rollin. *Life in Motion* (Portland, Ore.: Rudra Press, 1997).

[6] Speece, Conrad, and William Thomas Crow. *Ligamentous Articular Strain: Osteopathic Manipulative Techniques for the Body* (Seattle: Eastland Press, 2001).

[7] Ward, Robert, ed. *Foundations for Osteopathic Medicine,* 2nd ed. (Philadelphia: Lippincott Williams and Wilkins, 2003), 908.

[8] Comeaux, Zachary. *Robert Fulford, DO, and the Philosopher Physician* (Seattle: Eastland Press, 2002).

[9] Ward, Robert. Op. cit.

[10] Chila, Anthony. "To Know the Entirety of a Bone" (elective course workshop, AAO Convocation, Ottawa, Canada, AAO, Indianapolis, 2003).

[11] Chila, Anthony. "Rheumatoid Arthritis: A Connective Tissue Disease Process" (elective course workshop, AAO Convocation, Colorado Springs, AAO, Indianapolis, 2004).

[12] Tricot, Pierre. *Approche tissulaire de l'ostéopathie: un modèle du corps conscient* (Vannes cedex, France: Editions Sully, 2002).

Chapter 3

Vibration or Oscillation
in Osteopathic Thought

Vibratory Motion—A Subtle Trend

Vibration, or oscillation, has been used as a component of diagnosis and treatment in various forms since the beginning of osteopathy. Vibration has been included instinctively in the application of force considering rhythm as an aspect of motion. Additionally, vibration has had a special place in the development of an alternative cosmology in which the nature and state of the patient can be reinterpreted.

Combining these themes, this chapter follows the roots of vibration and oscillation in the philosophical milieu at the time of Still, Sutherland, and Fulford, with some reference to the influences on these three by Herbert Spencer and his student, Walter Russell. We will explore the specific application of the use of vibration and periodic motion in numerous contexts. We will then introduce the role of oscillatory processes in the further elucidation of the nature of somatic dysfunction and the neuromuscular physiological basis for explaining it using conventional science. In Chapter 8, we will significantly expand on this theme.

Rhythmic Osteopathy?

On the surface, rhythmic techniques of osteopathy do seem eccentric and representative of a philosophically insular approach, perhaps not really osteopathic manipulation at all. What makes a technique osteopathic? The current panoply of manipulative techniques developed largely from the objectification of the body as a machine, an analogy used frequently by Still, with parts to be adjusted by the active mechanic. The practitioner places the body of the patient, at rest, on a treatment table as if it were a machine that is temporarily turned off for a repair. This apparently challenges one to recall the unifying focus in theme and conviction of the founder, Dr. Still, that the person is a functional unity in a functional universe. He stressed both the material and vital basis of the person in his analogies of the Triune Man. The presuppositions of one's world view are rarely included in medical or health care discussions. They are implicit and largely contextual. And so we reconcile this rift between the material and the vital by simply stating that the "structure and function are *interrelated.*" However, we rarely explore the nature of this interrelationship beyond a very rudimentary level, partly due to the complexities involved, but also due to the general unfamiliarity with the method and value of philosophical concepts and reasoning.

The rest of this chapter reviews some of the essential elements of the osteopathic approach to the patient, including philosophical issues, and the appearance of vibratory or oscillatory methods used in the application of osteopathic philosophy by key members of the profession. In Chapter 8 we will address other aspects of this complexity in the interrelationship of structure and function under the more contemporary theme of energy medicine.

Intellectual Roots

The reader is asked to recall, or recognize, that Dr. Still rarely focused on teaching specific techniques. He felt that effective diagnosis and treatment were targeted at the root cause, not symptoms, of a loss of health. He focused on the practitioner's knowledge, observation, principle, and judgment to determine the nature of a treatment in the individual patient. He used whatever method worked, but his vision was directed toward a fuller, deeper understanding of the nature of the patient as a person. However, certain presuppositions, sometimes stated clearly and other times vaguely or not at all, created a context for understanding Still's statements.

Our first challenge today, in following the novelty of his approach, is to try to understand the full intent and implications of this approach. The further challenge then is to optimize the extent to which decisive information about the patient's state of being can be discerned through manual contact. Still's primary vehicle for teaching was the anatomy, which he described as the tangible evidence of the work of divine intent. Still's analogies were consistently driven by the idea of reading the orderliness of the Creator, and the patterns of body organization for health implied. Progressively, he attended to subtle, more profound patterns of organization of body function in the development of his thought.

As mentioned, Still's thought developed in a social context. As observed by Still's biographer, Carol Trowbridge, much of the underpinning for Still's philosophy was the thought of Herbert Spencer and the intellectual climate produced in America by Spencer's integrated approach to evolutionary biology and cosmology.[1]

Herbert Spencer (1820–1903), an English philosopher in the classical style, developed an organized body of work around a variety of themes of human knowledge, including biology and physics. In developing his systematic philosophy, Spencer held that the unifying principles defining existence involved the compounding of the rules of motion and force between all bodies—inert, organic, or social. Each creature existed in a state of interactive balance of physical forces with those around it and changed due to the absorption or dissipation of motion. He described all interaction using the laws of Newtonian kinetics. Interactions between two objects or beings consisted either of inertial contact or of gravitational interaction, usually an alternation between the two. Since all states of being represented intermediate positions between these two extreme conditions, all motion was considered rhythmic, reflecting the alternating gravitational attraction of an object between opposite extremes and the shifting of balance in attraction-repulsion between these opposites. The state of inertia of any object changed as the distance between bodies changed after contact.

From the ensemble of the facts as above set forth, it will be seen that rhythm results whenever there is a conflict of forces not in equilibrium. If the antagonist forces at any point are balanced, there is rest, and in the absence of motion there is of course no rhythm. But if, instead of a balance, there is an excess of force in one direction, then for that motion to continue uniformly in that direction, it is requisite that the moving matter should, not withstanding its unceasing change of place, present unchanging relations to the source of the force by which its motion is produced and opposed. This, however, is impossible. Every further transfer through space must alter the ratio between the force concerned—must increase or decrease the predominance of the one force over the other—must prevent the uniformity of movement. And if the movement cannot be uniform, then, in the absence of acceleration or retardation continued through infinite time and space (results which cannot be conceived), the only alternative is rhythm.[2]

Spencer's 500-page *First Principles* created a foundation for Still's description of the interrelationship between structure and function. Still would later describe his science of osteopathy as the relationship of mind, matter, and motion.

A more succinct statement, possibly more relevant to our current discussion, is the following:

Rhythm being manifested in all forms of motion, we have reason to suspect that it is determined by some primordial condition to action in general.[3]

Spencer claimed that a firm philosophical understanding of these rules of motion and physics was gained by observation of the natural world; by analogy he extended these rules as consistent operational principles affecting form and function of the individual, the evolution of species, and patterns for social behavior. Spencer's work was expanded in several directions, including the formation of an intellectual movement focused through the "Twilight Club," among whose American members were social leaders Oliver Wendell Holmes, Walt Whitman, Mark Twain, Andrew Carnegie, and John Burroughs. The purpose of the club was to contemplate and discuss solutions for the new (twentieth) century in face of a downward trend in civilization. If social and political solutions were not found, civilization was in its twilight before extinction. Spencer had considerable social and political impact, including influence on the osteopathic

profession particularly through Still's appreciation of the importance and attributes of motion in living systems.

Another Branch of the Tree

The vibrant energy of the establishment of an osteopathic profession and its early successes were a catalyst in the lives of many
people. Born in Scotland, John Martin Littlejohn was drawn to
this new approach to medicine. Initially coming as a patient,
he was soon engaged intellectually. A highly educated man,
grounded in physiology, Littlejohn saw implications for a fuller
understanding of the person in a way that Dr. Still felt challenged
his own vision. As a consequence, the two great thinkers eventually parted company. Part of this argument was Littlejohn's
recommendation of a fuller appreciation of the study of physiology in understanding health and disease. We can see now, over
time, that Littlejohn's approach to biomechanics and physiology
represented valuable insights.

> It is not correct to speak of the body as a machine, nor as a
> mechanism, unless we speak of it as a vital mechanism.
>   The basis of the vital functions of the body is the blood
> circulation and nerve force action.[4]

Littlejohn integrated an appreciation of rhythmicity into
osteopathic theory and practice in several ways, which we will
explore in a later chapter, especially as this work has been carried
forward by John Wernham.

Progression of Osteopathic Thought

Although Still's vision was to attend simultaneously to the complementary function of all aspects of the whole person, genera-

tionally there has been a shift of focus by his students from one subset of anatomical or physiological variables to another. Articular position, restriction of motion, functional dynamics, response to respiration, and an array of tender points reflecting symptoms have each taken their turn as the focus of diagnosis and treatment. The greater challenge is to attend to these aspects, but to appreciate them as part of a larger pattern of organization of the person, or even a universe.

The four summary principles from meetings in Kirksville (AAO 1954 Yearbook, pp. 50–52) in the 1950s, now popularly taught in many osteopathic schools, articulate among them the osteopathic interest in the interrelationship of structure and function. Much time is spent in modern osteopathic training in the sciences to elucidate structure (through anatomical studies) and function (through physiological studies), but less time is spent on focusing on the aspect of the interrelationship. There seems to be a bias against doing the hard work of thinking on this scale. This trend of focusing on specific aspects of bioscience as an array of isolated influences, parts, and problems to solve is neither unique to osteopathy nor to science in general, but represents a challenge to human perception in general.

Principles of Osteopathic Philosophy

1. The human being is a dynamic unit of function.

2. The body possesses self-regulatory mechanisms that are self-healing in nature.

3. Structure and function are interrelated at all levels.

4. Rational treatment is based on these principles.

From Glossary of Osteopathic Terminology, in Ward, *Foundations for Osteopathic Medicine,* p. 1242.

It is my view that this relationship of structure and function is reflected in the dynamic, as well as spatial, character of the parts and whole. The reaching of physiology beyond cellular and receptor models into the domain of proteomics as a way of describing tissue is a step in that direction. Corresponding effort in the direction describing anatomical micro-architecture as in the tensegrity models[5,6] and in neural function will help elucidate the relationship. The concept of vibratory or oscillatory assessment and intervention presents an occasion to apply this dynamical appreciation in the *living person.*

Sutherland

We have briefly mentioned W. G. Sutherland, DO. Sutherland's introduction and elaboration of the cranial model is one of the first attempts to recognize the intrinsic nature of rhythmic process, beyond the beating of hearts and filling of lungs. His thought went through a lifelong evolution, as he mulled over the root concepts of osteopathy and the nature of freedom and restriction of motion. Beginning with the concept of cranial artic-ular motion, he saw further implications in Still's attention to the potency of the central nervous system as part of endogenous motion.[7]

Still had seen the characteristic of the living organism as the infusion of an extraneous ethereal force into matter, to form what he called Biogen, consistent with classical theories of animism or vitalism. Sutherland was able to take this vital potency to the level of physiological theory, palpable diagnoses and facilitative treatment using the organizing concept of "the Tide."[8]

Early on he seemed to give this a physical substrate in the form of the cerebral spinal fluid (CSF), attempting to reconcile Still's vital-ism with conventional physiology. For many years he struggled, trying to overcome the incredulity of most of his professional colleagues regarding the very idea of cranial bone motion, and eventually settled on a relatively limited, though intricate model recorded by the Lippincotts and H. Magoun.[9]

However, as further elaborated later by Jealous and others cited below, this Tide was viewed as more than a hydraulic unfolding of the central nervous system (CNS) disseminated through peripheral tissue. It was not delimited by Sutherland's published physical definitions as he continued to reflect on its nature as a creative life force.

Sutherland, however, through introduction of attention to this rhythmic Tide, introduced the dimension of temporospatial organization with periodic character into the arena of freedom and/or restriction of motion, a conventional osteopathic concept. However defined, periodic fluctuation of the life force became the leading principle behind Sutherland's later work, principally in diagnosis. (We will return to Sutherland's important concepts later in this chapter.)

Rhythm in the Work of Other Still Students

Elmer Barber, DO, who wrote the first text on osteopathy in 1898,[10] mentioned vibration as a means to break up congestion and inflammation. The application of periodic mobilizing force is more directly expressed in the teachings of Littlejohn, and, although Littlejohn's focus is often represented as limited to articular correction, the maintenance of dysfunctional relationships is markedly dynamical.

In all adjustive movements it is necessary to overcome the passive resistance of inertia in the mechanics of the structures, and the resistance of muscular activities. In the former, the ligaments and cartilages are principally involved, assisted by the weight of the body and, in treatment the freest possible position of the body must be adopted. In the latter, posture may reduce the body to a state of relative inactivity, but it is essential to ask the patient to allow the body to remain passive assisted by distracting the patient's attention from the field of adjustment, by asking the patient to inhale and exhale freely. In the attempt to maintain the passive state the muscles all over the body should be relaxed: in the cervical region a series of gentle movements to the head and neck will generally produce sufficient relaxation to enable a rapid adjustive movement before the muscles have sufficient time to establish tension. In the dorsal and lumbar regions, the best method of relaxing muscles is the arm and leg leverage during which the adjustment is made, or immediately afterwards. The relaxed arm, or leg, represents a neutral state in the mobility of the body, and this is why we practically always use the arm and leg leverage in the correction of the dorsal and lumbar lesions.[11]

If one recalls that the emphasis here is on articular correction or adjustment, the coupled oscillatory motion becomes an essential part of loosening ligaments and normalizing muscle tone.

In discussing the integration of oscillation into the context of British osteopathy, especially the work passed through John Wernham, a surviving student of Littlejohn, Laurie Hartman, DO, made the following comment:

Harmonic motion in osteopathic treatment has been in existence from the earliest times. Still had many students, one of these was J. M. Littlejohn, the founder of the Chicago College of Osteopathic Medicine and the British School of Osteopathy in London. He taught several of my tutors, Wer-

nham, Hall, Middleton, Webster-Jones, Blagrave, Hardy, Stod-
dard and many others. They all used some form of harmonic
rocking and oscillating in their treatment patterns.[12]

We will describe the contemporary work of Wernham and
other intellectual descendants of Littlejohn's in Chapter 5.

Suffice it to say here that in Littlejohn's view, "relaxing the
muscles" is preparatory. Vibration is one part of this. Subse-
quently, Denslow demonstrated a concomitant sympathetically
driven hypertonia, or constant muscle tension, which seemed
to be part of maintaining the restricted motion characteristic of
somatic dysfunction otherwise known then as the osteopathic
lesion.[13] In this context, Littlejohn's application of oscillation
can easily be seen as an effort to overcome this sympathetically
driven muscle hypertonia.

Developments in Rhythmic Resistive Duction

The muscle energy model of diagnosis and treatment recognizes
muscle hypertonia, or increased muscle tension, as a primary
causative force in articular restriction of motion. T. J. Ruddy, DO,
one of the acknowledged sources of the thought that later blos-
somed as Muscle Energy Technique, used active repetitive motion
by the patient as a part of a treatment sequence. He described
his "Osteopathic Rhythmic Resistive Duction Therapy"[14] as a
guided rhythmic voluntary muscular contraction made by the
patient which is intended to restore normal muscle tone. Either
increased or decreased tone of musculature, when one considers
the reciprocal roles of agonist and antagonist muscles, is a characteristic of somatic dysfunction. A strategy evoking repetitive
contraction of the musculature attached to a restricted "unit"
during the direct treatment procedure was, among other effects,

intended to "engender normal afferent impulses to all nerve centers particularly the pre-motor cortical area for reestablishing normal muscle tone." The practitioner sets the pace by calling for contractions, usually about sixty per minute. In this model, the intent is to restore normal neurological balance, within the conceptualization of the neuromuscular system at the time. However, Ruddy introduces rhythmic activity, giving it a significant role in treatment.

Fred Mitchell converted this technique to an active oscillatory motion against constant patient contractive force to treat scalene tightness under the heading of Vibratory Isolytic Technique as a strategy of overcoming the myotactic reflex associated with somatic dysfunction by "possibly overwhelming the proprioceptive mechanism."[15]

Russell, Sutherland, and Fulford— Unpublished Collaboration

In the discussion of Sutherland, we have mentioned the importance of periodic motion in the tradition of Spencer and Russell. Robert Fulford was a recent osteopathic graduate when he accompanied Dr. Sutherland in the 1940s to collaborate with Walter Russell. Russell, a practical philosopher, saw the world in terms compatible with Sutherland's principles of palpating the life force as a way of working in complementary fashion with the Creator. Walter Russell, after Spencer, was the coordinator of the Twilight Club mentioned above. His cosmology began by saying that "The universe in its entirety is One thinking, living, breathing, pulsing universal being."[16]

Following the ideas of Spencer, his mentor, Russell expressed that being, motion, and thought were intertwined concepts and interactive forces. Russell held this philosophically; Sutherland saw it clinically. This reinforced Sutherland in the significance of the motion he had palpated, as an extension of an endowed vital process, associated with breathing. It underscored the integration of this respiration with participation in a larger dimension of life. Respiration became the Breath of Life, concomitant with Russell's description of the life force.

Russell's cosmology also included the Pythagorean concepts of universal harmonic and rhythmic influences in creation. He contemporized and extrapolated this to describe all interactions as having a common balanced electromagnetic aspect. With this line of thought he recognized the importance of rhythmic motion to all levels of life. Further, this could provide a basis for physiological induction of indigenous cyclic motion through intention. Rollin Becker, another student of Sutherland's, brought forth this more clearly. The French osteopathic scholar Francois Bel makes the case, by analyzing the chronological sequencing of expression of key concepts by Sutherland, for the influence of Russell on Sutherland's concepts.[17] Those interested in studying this further are advised to try to procure a copy of Russell's *The Universal One.*

This association of Russell and Sutherland, witnessed by the young Robert Fulford, had a formative influence on his thought. Other concepts of Russell's that later had influence on Fulford's practice included the idea that "Mind is the concept force of this created universe of form. Form in matter is the reflected expression of the concept force." Or "Matter is the substance of mind." Another was the concept of *balanced rhythmic interchange.* Russell used it in his cosmogony to describe interaction at all levels, while Fulford was later to apply it in clinical practice to coordinate the interaction of trauma, dysfunction, and treatment in the patient.[18]

While Sutherland included a place for intention, for the spiritual dimension and oscillatory diagnosis, he applied the concept of therapeutic vibration only in a confined field. In *Teachings in the Science of Osteopathy,* there is a sequence describing lymphatic mobilization with vibration:

> The physiologic emptying requires a gentle and rather unique siphoning process in the thoracic duct. This process can be assisted or facilitated by the use of feeling, seeing, thinking, and knowing fingers. This guidance varies from manual manipulation. During the application, fingers of one hand establish a contact over lymph nodes while a transmitted vibration is initiated through the other hand, which is placed on top of it. A quiet pause-rest should occur between applications. The first application is to the upper left thorax near the axilla. The second is done with a lift to the area above the receptaculum chyli. The third is at the great omentum, with a lift. The transmitted vibration initiates the siphoning process.[19]

After this exchange between Sutherland and Russell, there was a struggle among Sutherland's students as to whether to define the cranial concept in articular terms as was the pattern of Sutherland up until this point, or to look for an expanded concept based on Sutherland's implications. There were other issues involved, including many beyond the scope of this book. However, the former, the articular view, prevailed and Fulford's interest in oscillation became a semi-independent train of thought in cranial practice.

Fulford's Elaboration of the Role of Vibratory Motion

Fulford, even as a young person, had been looking for unifying concepts that would coordinate the various treatment approaches he had been taught. He intuited a connection between Russell's and Sutherland's periodic rhythms and wanted ways of amplifying the concept to assist patients while conserving his energy. He followed these themes of vibratory motion though a series of trials. His 1940s black bag included homeopathic remedies. (Homeopathic remedies are made potent by rhythmic vibration.) He also pursued a course of study with Randolph Stone, DO, who had traveled the Orient studying ayurvedic and other healing systems and translated the concepts into polarity therapy. Basically, this marked an attempt to balance the electromagnetics of patient and operator to enhance the energetic state of the patient using the Eastern model of meridians to describe the nature of man. Stone recognized Fulford as an astute and insightful student.[20]

Fulford identified Stone's power not so much in his conceptualization of the nature of the body; rather, "It was his voice." Apparently Stone had a deep resonance, which was commanding, projecting vibratory energy in his speech. However, in his manuals on polarity therapy, Stone also cited his use of gentle rhythmic pressure to enhance the return of body balance.[21]

In any case, prior to 1955 by apparent chance, Fulford received a mailing that advertised the Foredom Percussion Vibrator as a physical therapy adjunctive device. The device had been used in the field of pulmonary therapy to mobilize consolidated secretions. Fulford saw the brochure and he would recall in personal conversation, "This was exactly what I was looking for. My supervisor at Union Carbide would say, 'whenever you can, have a machine do your work for you, take advantage of it.'"

Beginning intuitively, Fulford felt this adjunctive device to be a more effective means of transmitting his therapeutic intention through the application of vibratory force. According to his mentors cited above, musculoskeletal restriction of motion existed first in the energetic or "ethric" body of the patient, which supported the physical body. The percussion perpendicular to the surface of the skin maximized the potential for the skin to act as a transducer of energy from the physician to patient. The physician's intention was amplified by the vibratory waves of the percussive vibration. As in any osteopathic manipulative treatment, the monitoring hand at a strategic location was used to assess and modulate the placement and speed of the vibration. In addition, the hand assessed the appropriate end point of treatment. Progressively through empirical trials, Fulford found associations between symptoms, personal history of trauma, and palpable subtle changes in the person that he reconceptualized as changes in the etheric or energetic body. These parameters could be palpated on or off the body. Clearly there were correlative findings in terms of tissue texture change and alteration of motion characteristics. However, Fulford's main criterion for evaluating success was his assessment of the state of the body in the "ethric" field, or energy dimension. The original impetus to think this way came from the work and writings of the neurophysiologist H. S. Burr, who described a measurable L-field (life field).[22] However, Fulford drew nuances from a variety of sources and adapted them to his model of work.

Fulford, drawing from other descriptions of this vitality, described the physical breath that is "The Breath," or Breath of Life. One can see the compatibility with Sutherland's expression of the Tide, or life force. Consistent with Eastern conceptualizations of pranic breathing, Fulford made a connection between diaphragmatic breathing and an energy exchange beyond what we commonly express as oxidation-reduction through alveolar exchange. His palpation of respiration evolved as a hybrid between the primary respiration of Sutherland and the polarity issues involved with Randolph Stone's thought. In any case, breathing had an energetic character that was part of assessing the well-being of the patient, and was affected by trauma and amenable to manipulative release. It had more significance than simple mechanical motion or exchange of gases.

Although sometimes construed to the contrary, Fulford's main interest was not with vibration per se but with enhancing freedom of function on all levels, using the energy state of the body as the vehicle for diagnosis and treatment. He used subtle touch, magnets, quartz crystals, and other means, correlated with intention, to intervene for healing. On several occasions late in life, Fulford read at meetings a position statement:

> The human body is composed of complex interflowing streams of moving energy. When these energy streams become blocked or constricted we lose the physical, emotional, and mental fluidity potentially available to us. If the blockage lasts long enough, the result is pain, discomfort, illness and distress.[23]

In a discussion following a demonstration of treatment using a Vogel cut crystal as an amplification device for vibratory treatment, Fulford was asked how this related to the study of osteopathy. His reply was, "How can you be successful without the knowledge of osteopathy for diagnosis?"[24]

The key to Fulford's methods was a view of the person as a dynamic system in which restriction of this dynamic process was responsible for loss of health, motion, and comfort. Restriction was not limited to material mechanics. In his thoughts we see the root ideas of Still, Sutherland, Spencer, Russell, and Stone. And although Fulford's system is somewhat elaborate, vibration takes on a new significance in the expression of osteopathic thought. A more complete description of Fulford's concepts and methods is available in my prior work.[25]

Summary

Rhythmic manual interventions sometime challenge bodyworkers who have a fixed focus on favorite methods since they expand on the mechanical interpretation of biophysics and include other knowledge about the nature of the patient in diagnosing and treating. Sometimes intuition and a desire to serve precede our ability to fully explain a technique. But this should not limit our clinical application of effective techniques in our will to heal.

This book is an effort to place rhythmic concepts in the context of the classical struggle of osteopathy, and other aspects of bodywork, to treat the dysfunctional component as an aspect of the whole person. But our view of the whole person is framed by our perception of the nature and laws of function of the universe. This dimension is not routinely taught in medical school or other health care education but is clearly an aspect of Still's thoughts and is implicated in the work of many of his serious students.

> The Osteopath finds here the field in which he can dwell forever. His duties as a philosopher admonish him, that life and matter can be united, and that union cannot continue with any hindrance to free and absolute motion.[26]

The process of elucidating this quest did not begin or end with Still. From his predecessors (as represented in Spencer, in which rhythm is a necessary characteristic of all motion)[27] to his students through several generations (including Littlejohn, Sutherland, Becker, and Fulford), observation, diagnosis, and treatment may include this rhythmic aspect of motion. The use of rhythmic motion to diagnose and treat, and the desire to understand this relationship more fully, are embedded in the context of osteopathic tradition and thought and its current expression. They are also embedded in other traditions of bodywork, as will be discussed in Chapter 6.

References

[1] Trowbridge, Carol. *Andrew Taylor Still 1828–1917* (Kirksville, Mo.: The Thomas Jefferson University Press, 1991).

[2] Spencer, Herbert. *First Principles,* 5th ed. (New York: A. L. Burt Publishers, 1880), 220, 221. Originally published in 1864.

[3] Ibid., 234.

[4] Littlejohn, John Martin. Unpublished course notes transcribed by Lawrence Meyran (Archives, European School of Osteopathy, Maidstone, England, n.d.).

[5] Ingber, Donald. "Mechanobiology and diseases of mechanotransduction," *Annals of Medicine* 35(8), 2003, 564–577.

[6] Ho, Mae Wen. *The Rainbow and the Worm: The Physics of Organisms* (Singapore: World Scientific Publishing Co., 1998).

[7] Still, Andrew. *Philosophy and Mechanical Principles of Osteopathy* (Kirksville, Mo.: Osteopathic Enterprises, 1986), 44ff. Originally published in 1892.

[8] Sutherland, William. *Contributions of Thought* (Dallas: The Sutherland Cranial Teaching Foundation, 1967), 142ff.

[9] Magoun, Harold. *Osteopathy in the Cranial Field* (Kirksville, Mo.: Journal Printing Co, 1976).

[10] Barber, Elmer. *Osteopathy Complete* (Virginia Beach: Lifeline Press, 1889).

[11] Littlejohn, John Martin. *The Fundamentals of Osteopathic Technique* (Maidstone, England: Institute of Classical Osteopathy, n.d.), 98–99.

[12] Hartman, Laurie. Personal communication, 1998.

[13] Denslow, John, in Beal Myron. ed. *Selected Papers of John Stedman Denslow, D.O. Yearbook* (Indianapolis: American Academy of Osteopathy, 1993), 19ff.

[14] Ruddy, T. J. "Osteopathic Rhythmic Resistive Duction Therapy," *Yearbook* (Academy of Applied Osteopathy, 1961), 58–68.

[15] Mitchell, Fred. *The Muscle Energy Manual,* vol. 2 (East Lansing, Mich.: MET Press, 1995), 94.

[16] Russell, Walter. *The Universal One* (Waynesboro, Va.: University of Science and Philosophy, 1926), 2.

[17] Bel, Francois. "W. G. Sutherland a-t-il été influencé par Walter Russell?" *ApoStil, Le journal de l'Académie d'Ostéopathie,* March 2000, 14–22.

[18] Ibid.

[19] Sutherland, William. *Teachings in the Science of Osteopathy,* Anne Wales, ed. (Dallas: Sutherland Cranial Teaching Foundation, 1990), 136.

[20] Stone, Randolph. Unpublished letters to R. Fulford, 1955–1962.

[21] Stone, Randolph. *Wireless Anatomy of Man, Book II,* reprinted in *Polarity Therapy,* vol. 1 (Sebastopol, Calif.: CRCS Publications, 1986), 31.

[22] Burr, Harold S. *Blueprint for Immortality: The Electric Patterns of Life* (Essex, England: Saxton Walden, 1972).

[23] Fulford, Robert. *Vibrating Energy,* AAO Convocation presentation, 1992, personally transcribed notes, represented in Comeaux, 2002 (note 25, below).

[24] Ibid.

[25] Comeaux, Zachary. *Robert Fulford, DO, and the Philosopher Physician* (Seattle: Eastland Press, 2002).

[26] Still, Andrew. *Philosophy of Osteopathy* (Indianapolis: American Academy of Osteopathy, 1977), 197. Originally self-published in Kirksville, Mo., 1899.

[27] Spencer, Herbert. Op. cit.

Chapter 4

American Integration of Rhythmic Motion

Basic Osteopathy and Osteopathy in the Cranial Field

It should be clear from the preceding chapter that the use of oscillation or vibration, although not a primary theme in American osteopathic practice, has been a recurrent theme among important reflective or intuitive DOs. The majority of the examples of the use of integration of rhythmic procedures in manual medicine, known to the author, have been in the osteopathic context. Later in this chapter, examples from several other bodywork practice traditions will be described.

As mentioned several times already, in Still's and Sutherland's writings the influence of Spencer and Russell, with their inclusion of the ontogenic role (referring to a state of *being*) of oscillation, are subtle but present. Their teaching reflects a philosophical world view in which the physics of motion is inherently periodic or rhythmic by its nature. However, it has been suggested that several of Sutherland's key phrases were derived or adapted from contact with Walter Russell. We will further discuss this influence when we describe how Dr. Fulford adapted Sutherland's teachings derived from Russell. In osteopathy in the cranial field, progressive theory and research continue to elaborate an explanation of Dr. Sutherland's observations of inherent body rhythmicity.

Appreciating rhythmic motion as part of diagnosis has been a primary part of the work of Sutherland and his students since the beginning. Sutherland refers to this rhythmic motion as respiration, primary or secondary, since respiration was a recognized rhythmic function of the body. It is his plea for equal recognition of the physiologically integral role of cranial mobility and the force that it represents.

Fulford's Energetic Model— Beyond the Cranial Model

As mentioned above, one of Sutherland's students, Robert Fulford, amplified the significance of the rhythmic aspect of nature, physics, and the person. Proposing an additional energetic dimension to fascia, he coached his students to understand the patient, looking beyond biomechanical parts and the way in which they might interact in the context of Newtonian physics. He reread the physiology and anatomy he had been taught through a filter of bioenergetic medicine, more compatible with a quantum physics world view. This was a challenge in his day since that type of formulation or modeling had scarcely been done in manual medicine or bodywork.

Though rarely expressed in this way outside of Still's writing, the osteopathic definition of the person is the key to osteopathic science. Dr. Still encouraged his students to bring philosophy into clinical practice. Following his inclination, Robert Fulford reevaluated the nature of the person and developed an energetic concept of the person and further developed various effective amplifications of manipulation, including percussion vibration.

In this context, a fuller functional concept of a person included integrated but overlapping levels of activity, or complexity, contributing to the constitution of the person. Whereas A. T. Still had variously outlined the human body as a constellation of systems (vascular, neural, and so on) and again as "body, mind, and spirit," then later as matter and biogenic force, Fulford took another approach. Following the suggestions of Harvard neurologist H. S. Burr, he postulated that besides the physical body as typically understood in biological science, the person's body participated in or emanated an energy field, or L-field (life field). Later, following description in Eastern spirituality and esoteric healing models, he called this the etheric or "ethric" body or field. In either case it was an operational vibratory phenomenon.

Redefining Dysfunction

Corresponding to this level of function, this etheric or energy body played as much a part in everyday strains and bruises of the body of a person as does the molecular level of organization in body tissues. Tissue had a memory both molecular as well as in the etheric field or body. This was analogous to the impact of a collision on the metal (or fiberglass) on our automobile fenders. Impacts leave a memory due to the plasticity of the medium experiencing the force resulting in deformation. In living tissue, Fulford termed this distortion of the connective tissue matrix that resulted from trauma an "energy sink."

Let me describe the contextual meaning for the term *sink*. For those unfamiliar with this term, it is borrowed from soldering, a process of joining two pieces of metal. The solder, which is intended to bond the two pieces together, is itself a metal that liquifies at a relatively low temperature. It is applied heated in the liquid state to the edges of each of the two pieces intended to be joined; the heating instrument is withdrawn, and the solder cools and solidifies, binding the two pieces together. If a third metal element is to be joined within a short distance of this bond, we can repeat the process. However, if a sufficient amount of the heat energy involved in making this new bond reaches the previously completed joint, the latter will come apart as its solder melts again. To avoid this problem, the craftsman will clamp a removable piece of metal between these two union points which will absorb any excess heat transmitted from the new work site. This clamp, which absorbs or drains and retains energy, is commonly called a *sink*.

Fulford analogized from this example, describing the tissue memory of trauma, which made itself known through the physical symptoms of pain or restriction of motion as an energy sink. The energy sink, as a form of dysfunction, represented a decreased level of endogenous rhythmic oscillation, a dampening of inherent vibration, as it were, in response to the devitalizing shock of trauma. This phenomenon existed in the etheric or energetic body, or electromagnetic field of the person. Often, especially in complex or treatment-resistance cases, the answer was to be found in resolving the dysfunction at this level.

In this context Fulford added another dimension to our modeling of the connective tissue matrix, the fascia, amplifying the significance of how this medium recorded traumatic impact:

> When trauma strikes (physical or emotional), the electric field of the fascia is shocked into a sink. ... We can substitute the word fascia for the word field: then we have a better understanding of the process.[1]

In describing the activity of tissue in energy terms, Fulford intended to amplify the descriptions of structures and functions characteristically described in anatomy, physiology, and biochemistry with this sense of the etheric body. He conceived the etheric body to be a further layer of organization of protoplasm, like a glove over a hand, with vibration as its normal integrative activity. This dimension or layer of organization did not necessarily contradict or dismiss any of the conventional teaching in the biological, medical, or osteopathic sciences. Rather, it complemented them, represented an additional level of understanding of the nature of the person, and added another dimension to include in history, physical examination, and treatment.

With this extended conceptualization of health and disease, some of the more chronic causes of pain, deformity, and distress could be further explained. The energy body participated in physical, emotional, and spiritual experience. The source of trauma, as in an auto accident, may have been exclusively physical. Or it may have been a mix of components. Later, the residual dysfunction associated with whiplash strain, after normal tissue healing has occurred, may be due to the unattended results of the emotional energetic aspect of the initiating event. In the auto accident example, the emotional component might include the fear in anticipation of the impact, the unresolved anger at the perpetrator, or a continued feeling of vulnerability. Additionally, the injury sustained might initially be totally of an emotional or spiritual nature, as the etheric, emotional, and spiritual bodies of the individual were viewed as concentrically higher forms of existence.[2,3]

This view of the constitution of the person opened up another possible level of interpersonal contact and relationship in both everyday experience and in therapeutic contact. The impact of words, intentions, and interpersonal gestures had a particular importance, since they are the currency of interpersonal exchange on the emotional and spiritual level. Fulford would often cite that "thoughts are things"; in addition to their capacity to harm, they can convey the intentions of a healer and in this way may be as important as his or her manual contact.

In this train of thought, unresolved trauma may be due to the thoughts, attitudes, or actions of others important to the patient —a parent or spouse, for example. And since the relationship of parent and child begins with conception, pre-birth or birth-related trauma, including emotional, might underlie congenital or unresolving symptoms or conditions.

To work in this context, Fulford cultivated a climate of kindness and gentleness and introduced restorative vibratory force in several ways. He began with attention to the basic concepts and rhythms of cranial osteopathy, but he felt this was part of a bigger picture. Initially, his additional application of vibration was through homeopathic (succussed) remedies and Bach flower remedies. Next he was to maximize the endogenous rhythm of breathing through special exercises. Still further, as mentioned above, at least by 1955 he began using the Foredom Percussion Vibrator, which he used until his death. In the 1960s Fulford began using a refined, polished quartz crystal, in the style of Marcel Vogel, to amplify his healing intention. Just as crystals were earlier used as transducers of radio waves, he used them to modulate both his intention and the patient's vital energy. Additionally, at times he would use the electromagnetic influence of simple bar magnets.

Redefining Treatment

For practicality, Fulford developed his treatment into a general protocol in the context of which the particular dysfunctions of the patient would be discovered and addressed. However, at times he would directly focus on the region of primary concern to the patient or himself with intention and vibratory force. Tissue resonance, harmony in the etheric field, and enhanced natural respiration were used as indicators that treatment was improving the health of the individual.

In a typical treatment session after a known trauma, a history and physical exam would be followed by evaluation of the area of interest. If he appreciated a deficit in vibratory character, manual contact would be applied with or without the assistance of the percussion vibrator. The latter would be used over a bony prominence to maximize the dissemination of vibratory wave force through the soft tissue of the region treated. For example, treatment of the pelvis and lower lumbar area would include vibration applied to the greater trochanter, at the upper femur. The transmitted vibration would be appreciated by a "listening" hand at the opposite side of the pelvis. Experience would guide with regard to frequency and amount of pressure and duration.

The current context cannot give all the details of diagnosis and treatment and Fulford's many discursive thoughts and influence. Those who want more are referred to Dr. Fulford's *Touch of Life*, which Fulford wrote with the assistance of a ghostwriter as a book for the general public. Also of interest may be my *Robert Fulford, DO, and the Philosopher Physician,* written after his death. As an understudy of Fulford's for years, I also had opportunity to review Dr. Fulford's reading piles, personal files, and notebooks, at the request of his family, as they were collected from his study.[4]

Other American Rhythmic Approaches— Ruddy and Mitchell

As introduced in the history described in Chapter 2, T. J. Ruddy, DO, used oscillatory motion in his treatment of restriction of motion. Ruddy would diagnose using the criteria of his day and treat with repetitive isolytic voluntary contractions. This systematic use of rhythmic motion was intended to restore normal function. Ruddy, a student of Still, appreciated the importance of vascular nutrition for muscle and the reciprocal contraction of muscle to promote circulation. He described the state of dysfunction with strain or trauma:

Each muscle involved in the restricted movements of a single vertebra becomes weakened through lack of motion, essential to its own blood supply. Tone diminishes and though manipulation to mobilize the vertebra and its embedding soft tissue is administered, until the muscle is reconditioned to normal tone and contraction the freedom of fluid flow is obstructed, and in turn the effected lesioned rib movements tend toward chronicity.[5]

In Ruddy's view, articular dysfunction limits nutrition to muscle, and leads to atony or weakening of muscle. Manipulation is not complete until the muscle is reconditioned. This is the intended role of his resistive duction technique. It is described as having five steps:

The technique of employment of rapid rhythmic resistive muscle contraction is simple:

1. Resist the levers to which the contracting muscle is attached.
2. Patient contracts the muscle repeatedly, synchronous with the pulse rate and faster to double the pulse rate or higher, counting one-two, two-two, three-two, up to ten-two, the frequency at the close to be five-two in five seconds, if not an acute painful movement.
3. Press the part to be moved aiding the contracting muscle.
4. Counter pressure on the part articulating with the restricted unit.
5. Employ skeletal muscle contraction to pump visceral circulation.[6]

The stated purpose is again clarified to be an increase in the speed and strength of blood flow to tissue to ensure cellular nutrition, to recondition individual muscle fascicles, and to reinitiate normal neural impulses to reestablish muscle tone.

Key features of the method are the intent to induce tissue nutrition through rhythmic muscle contraction. The contractions are localized by focal hand contacts by the physician. However, the contractions are active voluntary contractions by the patient.

Following Ruddy, Fred Mitchell, Sr., developed the idea of correction of restriction through what he terms isolytic rhythmic resistance. This method has been described elsewhere as Muscle Energy Technique.[7]

The Next Generation

The current generation of students of Still, Sutherland, and Fulford has the challenge of sorting this out and deciding how to take the work further into a synthetic model of manual work, sometimes called the expanded osteopathic concept.

Carlisle Holland, DO, who has done considerable work in applying cranial osteopathy to children, has utilized the percussion vibrator (the "hammer," as Fulford sometimes called the vibrator) as a device to create an opportunity for connective tissue release. As an extension of cranial and connective tissue conceptualizations of the body, he uses one or more machines in resonant or dissonant fashion. The vibratory force is envisioned as remobilizing adherent fascial planes after traumatic restriction. Importance is paid to the energetic nature of the body in maintaining its form, including connective tissue arrangements. Another level of vibratory work is that of thought and Holland describes the relationship of transference between patient and practitioner.

Rajiv Yadava, DO, continued for some time to teach the course in which he assisted Dr. Fulford during the last several years of his life. The emphasis is primarily preservationist, to my understanding.

John McPartland, DO, and Eric Mein, MD, have applied the principles of entrainment of harmonic oscillators as an explanation for our ability to influence the cranial rhythmic impulse of patients as treated in Sutherland's cranial model. They review the hypotheses put forth to explain the intrinsic motility of the brain, make note of other biological oscillatory functions and phenomena in the body, and hypothesize that "the CRI is the perceptible entrainment, a palpable harmonic frequency of multiple biologic oscillators." Further: "Our entrainment hypothesis may also explain how CST [craniosacral treatment] practitioners bring about therapeutic changes in the patients." They develop the theme of coupled oscillation as a phenomenon in nature and its applicability to operator-patient interaction.[8]

Kenneth Nelson and colleagues have used the model of the Traube-Haering-Meyer wave, a partially understood but generally recognized physiological phenomenon, to validate and demonstrate the relationship of the cranial rhythm to other observable body rhythms.[9]

James Jealous, DO, elaborates a history of Sutherland's appreciation and description of the oscillatory aspect of biological processes in a person. He uses, as Fulford did, the interrelated concepts of the Tide and the Breath of Life, with deeper significance, as avenues for diagnosis and treatment. Again, the means of engagement is through synchrony with endogenous rhythmic motion. As with Sutherland, the means of intervention is manual, but augmented by a shift of attention and loving intention, as with Fulford. The perceptible movement is considered significant beyond the mechanical and includes dimensions that are vitally transcendental, spiritual, and in any case more sublime than the physical, biomechanical dimension alone. Diagnosis and treatment are guided by the practitioner trying to find and free the "health" of the individual.

Through transmutation of forces, manual contact in the context of loving intention can induce clinical improvement. Clinical effectiveness is increased by attending to the Long Tide, an oscillatory dynamic with characteristic base rate of one cycle each 2 to 3 minutes. As noted above, this approach integrated the osteopathic emphasis of treating according to one's progressively refined appreciation of the nature of the person, beginning with embryogenesis.[10] These and other aspects are taught under the umbrella of the biodynamic model.

I, Zachary Comeaux, teach a course in Fulford's synthetic methods. The key to this presentation is the integration of physiology with the apparently more esoteric aspects of energetic bodywork, including Fulford's osteopathic expression. Based on an in-depth review of Fulford's source material as well as intimate contact with the doctor, the course attempts to explicate what Dr. Fulford did not say through his terse papers and cryptic comments. Fidelity to the spirit of Fulford's work is preserved while integrating concepts from neurophysiology as well as Zen and other Eastern approaches to management of attention and action.

The concepts and methods described in this book as Facilitated Oscillatory Release (FOR) evolved out of this effort to explore, evaluate, and evolve Dr. Fulford's synthesis. This prospect was discussed with Fulford and received his approval. FOR will be explored in more depth after further development of supportive data and concepts in Part II of this book.

Incidentally, there are recognized commonalities with other approaches, especially Wernham's application of the teachings of Littlejohn. This material came to my attention after beginning the FOR endeavor. As a result there are unique features that evolved from the desire to apply Fulford's amplification methods and philosophy of the nature of the patient without the availability of a percussion vibrator, crystal, or other device. The approach includes considerations for treating trauma involving multiple planes of body organization. To further elucidate the structural-functional interrelatedness of the person, additionally, I am involved in biophysiological research to demonstrate the compatibility of the energetic or vibratory approach to somatic dysfunction and newer conceptualization in the field of neurobiology of oscillatory function. These include the concept of central pattern generations and resonant cell assembly models for explaining the binding and coding of perceptual experience. Application to the peripheral nervous system may clarify the nature of postural as well as proprioceptive patterns of muscular coordination and dysfunction. Numerous investigators implicate temporospatial coding as the primary means of internal communication within the neuromuscular system. This complements the classical view of coordination through a network of pathways, ganglia, and nuclei. A fuller discussion of this area is the topic of Chapter 8. Practical applications of these oscillatory events may help further define the functional nature of the person and clarify our understanding of dysfunction in the style of investigation such as by Still and others, as elaborated above.

The work of Milton Trager, stemming from a different line of thought entirely, involved the use of rhythmic motions. This approach will be described in Chapter 6. The originality of this intuitive and creative line of self-directed work is exciting.

References

[1] Fulford, Robert. *Are We On the Path? The Collected Works of Robert C. Fulford, DO,* T. Cisler, ed. (Indianapolis: The Cranial Academy, Inc., 2003).

[2] Bailey, Alice. *Esoteric Healing* (New York: Lucis Publishing Co, 1953).

[3] Johnston, Brenda. *New Age Healing* (Sussex, England: self-published, 1975).

[4] Comeaux, Zachary. *Robert Fulford, DO, and the Philosopher Physician* (Seattle: Eastland Press, 2002).

[5] Ruddy, T. J. "Osteopathic Rhythmic Resistive Duction Therapy," *Yearbook* (Academy of Applied Osteopathy, 1961), 58–68.

[6] Ibid.

[7] Mitchell, Fred. *The Muscle Energy Manual,* vol. 2 (East Lansing, Mich.: MET Press, 1995), 94.

[8] McPartland, John, and Eric Mein. "Entrainment and the Cranial Rhythmic Impulse," *Alternative Therapies,* 3(1), 1997, 40–45.

[9] Nelson, Kenneth, Nicette Sergueef, and Thomas Glonek. "Cranial Manipulation Induces Sequential Changes in Blood Flow Velocity on Demand," *American Academy of Osteopathy Journal,* 14(3), 2004, 15–17.

[10] Jealous, James. *Emergence of Originality: A Biodynamic View of Osteopathy in the Cranial Field* (Franconia, N.H.: self-published, n.d.).

Chapter 5

European Osteopathic Rhythmic Methods

Littlejohn's and Wernham's Preservation of Rhythmic Technique

The father of European osteopathy is also the father of European osteopathic rhythmic methods. John Martin Littlejohn, with the experience as dean of the American School of Osteopathy and the Chicago College of Osteopathy, returned to Britain and in 1917 founded the British School of Osteopathy. Littlejohn stressed the importance of physiology in addition to biomechanics, which was one of his falling-out points with Dr. Still. In a paper alleged to be his, Littlejohn describes the importance of rhythmicity in osteopathic work.[1]

One of Littlejohn's students, John Wernham (1906–2007), dedicated his life to the furtherance of his master's concepts and methods. Operating as the Institute of Classical Osteopathy beginning in 1954, Wernham continued to practice and teach into his ninety-ninth year. Reorganizing and publishing much of Littlejohn's work, Wernham[2] distributed a description largely reflecting Littlejohn's views on rhythm in osteopathy from the above cited paper. In this small work, the notation is made by Littlejohn of the gross physiological rhythmic processes of respiration and cardiac function. The importance of correcting spinal vertebral lesions whose corresponding nerve supply included these vital organs (the main point of the Littlejohn paper) is covered. In addition, he makes note that since rhythmic process is universal in the body, in one sense all dysfunction represents an arrhythmia.

> The World of Rhythm—Here we have a world of processes underlying all body activity, gross and subtle. There are loco-motion, mastication, respiration, peristalsis, etc., together with nerve oscillation, enzyme reaction, hormone secretion, etc. In health, the rhythm flows unnoticed, but if there is a break in the coordinated function or the structural integrity of the organism, then the disturbance is made manifest.[3]

Littlejohn intended these insights to encourage a person to have a deeper appreciation for the value of osteopathy as a healing science. Treatment of arrhythmias in this publication involved focusing on the specific spinal levels involved in sympa-thetic supply to the appropriate tissue, as described by Littlejohn. These focal lesions would receive special emphasis in a general treatment protocol, as will now be described.

Wernham's methods routinely incorporate gentle rhythmic articular mobilization. For a long period of his teaching life, Wernham popularized this approach as the General Osteopathic Technique, or GOT. The protocol has now been termed osteopathic body adjustment, implying that it is the one true way to practice. It covers spine, rib cage and extremities, systematically assessing restriction and mobilizing with articulation, gentle compressive swaying, or rotation of the torso. The cervical spine is treated with a regional rotational thrust. In the context of this general technique, relative segmental or focal restrictions of motion are discovered and mobilized by rhythmically accentuating the usual form used in diagnostic motion challenge.

Although treated several times by Mr. Wernham, I have abstracted most of the description of this treatment approach from a video presentation.[4]

In this method, the practitioner applies rhythmic articulation to the spine in several positional phases. Initially, evaluation begins with observation, and then noting the response to a gentle rhythmic sidebending motion challenge. Following treatment to the spine in a seated position, the practitioner treats the supine patient, first on the right side then left side of the body, followed by the lower then the upper extremities. The motions are smoothed and strengthened by the embracing support of the practitioner, who engages and moves the treated member in a gentle but firm manner. Movements are methodical, slow, and decisive. Circumduction of the left lower extremity begins to engage the lumbar vertebrae. Still supine, the patient receives regional thrust with rotational motion, then fine tuning with gentle translational motion.

Next, the practitioner has the patient lie prone with the knees flexed and applies rhythmic connective tissue release to the pelvis and lower limbs from the feet. Long lever circumduction of the right then left sides of the body persistently looks for areas of remaining restriction and softens the spinal curves. Paravertebral tissues are released using the rocked pelvis to transmit motion. Progressively, just as a likeness gradually appears among the daubs of paint on an artist's canvas, total body adjustment recreates normalcy in a strained body through a methodical application of rhythmic force.

As the protocol progresses, the patient is treated in a side-lying position with the top leg held off table and torsional rocking is applied through the shoulders. A supine "dog" technique is added before having the patient sit for a side-to-side oscillatory rocking again with wise searching fingers looking to direct force through stiff areas of the spine and rib cage. The treatment concludes with a spinal traction tug with bilateral underarm contact.

The individual maneuvers are intended to have local, regional, and whole-body effects. The rhythmic movements are gentle, almost in the form of a dance, despite the fact that some of the distension and excursion takes fascia and joints to the potentially restrictive barrier.

In Wernham's teaching, rhythmic motions are not the key feature. They represent a tactical means of gentle articulation around what are described as mini-fulcra that have the additive effect of mobilizing the whole body. Since the body is living tissue, specific joint mobilization at the site of symptoms, including pain, is not the successful strategy. The emphasis is on treating the whole body, "giving it back to itself," as Wernham quotes Littlejohn, and in so doing, engaging the local lesion or restriction back into a pattern of total body unified, integrated function. This return of mobility or stabilized physiologically integrated motion is required to cure a vital system such as the body.

Rhythm is used because "the body is a rhythmic structure and we are trying to impose rhythm where it does not exist," i.e., the lesioned area. With the extremities, circumduction is used because "the body moves in circles." And so rhythmic motion is recognized as acceptable to the body; it is gentle, and achieves the goal of reintegrating function in a manner the body accepts. We will discuss this under the topic of rhythmic entrainment in a theoretical section in Chapter 8.

Having experienced it, I will attest to the effectiveness of this application of rhythmic force. The question remains as to how to integrate the benefits of the technique into other routines without weakening the effect of treatment. Wernham disparaged neuromuscular and eclectic techniques as violating the philosophy of treating the whole integrated person by attempting a shortcut that leads to short-term improvement but no long-lasting cure. "You cannot break osteopathy into parts," he commented. There is a philosophic bias or stance here about what constitutes the relationship between the specific complaint and the unity of total body function. Others obviously see other solutions to this dilemma. A suggested method for accommodating the benefits of gentle rhythmic articulation, and other dimensions of impact, will be discussed under the topic of Facilitated Oscillatory Release in Part II.

Harmonic Technique

Similar mobilization has intuitively been included in the repertoire of many British osteopaths but finds an organized presentation as a separate modality in the Harmonic Therapy or Harmonic Technique described by Laurie Hartman, DO, and Eyal Lederman, DO.[5] Lederman has spent a considerable part of his professional life reflecting on and expressing the physiological principles by which osteopathic manipulation works.[6]

This theme carried over heavily into his description of Harmonic Technique.[7] Application of the rhythmic protocols to an individual patient requires an appreciation of the characteristics of harmonics in physics and the extension of these to tissue behavior.

The first principle to be understood in this area of biophysics is that under stress, connective tissue distorts or changes shape. In Lederman's description, articular ligaments and joint capsules are examples of connective tissue responding in such a manner. Recall that from our discussion of connective tissue above that certain principles apply.

Routine distention of tissue in its elastic range is due to alterations in the amorphous matrix or ground substance. Such deformational change will usually return to more normal, resting length since the potential bond energy is conserved in the tissue.[8] However, recurrent strain, as in overuse syndrome, may result in fibrin buildup to reinforce native tissue where increased demand requires increased strength to limit further injury. In so doing, articular mobility may be compromised.

Additionally, the natural healing process may result in fibrin production, which also limits some aspect of joint, vascular, or nerve function. A focal example of this is persistent inflammation (healing activity) associated with the joint capsule or synovial lining of a joint. Although the physiological intent is joint protection, exaggerated healing may limit proper function by creating a restriction of motion or pain.

In designing an intervention to restore normal motion, the parameters of normal motion must be understood. In natural motion, on many levels, rhythmicity is a key feature. Repetition conserves energy in elastic tissues to be used in the next cycle. Each organ or tissue conserves energy operating on it and through it by rhythmic stretch to conserve potential energy and rhythmic release of this energy. Conservation of energy in the reciprocating activities of gait (arm swing, leg swing, torso torsion) is a primary example of this phenomenon.

In this regard, the concept of tissue resonance is also a key function. Each tissue in the body (with a focus here on the tissue supporting the joints) has its native resonant frequency, that frequency at which minimal energy is dissipated by the tissue and the maximum is made available for continued work. To analogize to an old wind-up clock, this characteristic causes the tissue to behave much like springs as the limbs behave as pendulums in expressing rhythmicity in function.

Body members possess mass. The center of mass of one body part or region may create a balance counterforce when an opposing motion occurs in another direction. If this motion becomes rhythmically repetitive, we call the two cyclically operating units coupled oscillators. In locomotion, limbs and trunk regions operate as freely oscillating coupled masses enabling energy-efficient linear displacement of the body. A center of mass, such as the pelvis, lower extremity, or upper extremity, assumes a role as a repetitive oscillator to conserve the potential energy of an action, once initiated, on its way to completion. As such, one step forward creates an inertial state on which the next step uses the conserved energy stored in the joint and other tissues of the body to proceed with less effort.

Each freely oscillating mass relies on coordinated but coupled counter movement from another part of the system to turn the rotational and counter-rotational movements into purposeful linear displacement. And so, the toe off of one gait cycle creates a base on which the swing forward phase of the opposing lower limb can carry the body forward, while the torsion of the trunk and the opposed momentum of arm swing creates a system of balanced, coupled oscillators that create smoothly coordinated locomotion while maintaining balance and conserving energy.

In this conservation system, each tissue starts at a resting length and has a range of free motion during which recovery of resting length is assured. This is the elastic range of tissue distortion in which the elastic loading serves to store potential energy. It is readily reversible with removal of load. If the trauma or strain exceeds the force limits capable of absorption in this elastic range, plastic deformation of the tissue fibers may make repair or return of normal function more complex and may dampen the natural resonance of the tissue.

These principles of resonance, and elastic and plastic deformation of tissue, may be used to therapeutic advantage after injury. In so doing, an external force is applied to restore the resting length and the natural harmonic resonance. To do so the operator must appropriately assess the degree and location of compromise, and externally apply energy to correctively deform the damaged tissue, to coax it back into natural conformation and functional resonance.

As with Wernham, Lederman's description of principles and techniques offers a framework from which to begin diagnosing and treating these injuries. Lederman includes a brief section on oscillatory stretch consistent with Littlejohn, as quoted at the beginning of this chapter. First, he describes the concept of hysteresis and principles of treatment involving the parameters of loading force and duration in stretch. He then describes cyclic stretching in which the force applied in each cycle is small (compared to an equivalently effective constant stretch), but with significant cumulative effect. The first four cycles of a stretching to 10 percent beyond the muscles' resting length are found to produce 80 percent of the length change expected.[9]

As the reader will later appreciate, there is a considerable amount of common ground between Harmonic Technique and Facilitated Oscillatory Release, so much so, that when I discovered this line of thought, I was thrilled at the reinforcement of my own insight but reticent to be influenced too soon by this train of thought. Too many details needed to be explored independently for clarity of the FOR approach. Two of the main areas of difference between the two treatment models are the way in which the neuroregulatory system is engaged and the manner of localization of tissue restriction of motion.

Regarding the engagement of the neuroregulatory system, in Lederman's model it is recognized that the hypertonia of muscle supporting a joint may, after trauma, restrict motion of the joint. It is recognized by many[10,11] that the complex coordinative roles of the alpha and gamma motor system (the muscle spindle system) probably contribute significantly to this hypertonia. Lederman makes the assumption here and in *Fundamentals of Manual Therapy* that the quiescence of the gamma motor system during passive manipulation implies that there is minimal effect on the system at this point. He then recommends a combination of patient rhythmic resistant activity during externally applied oscillation as the optimal treatment method. This is consistent with but does not cite the exercise protocols of Giselher Schalow, now gaining recognition in rehabilitative medicine circles.[12] I see the afferent input of oscillation by either method as having theoretical benefit and effect by means described in Part II.

As the reader will see in Chapter 8, there may be an extended role for the muscle spindle and other neuroregulatory components in the process of natural and dysfunctional postural, proprioceptive balance, especially as related to rhythmic afferent input.

In Lederman's text, he cites as major mechanisms the complementarity and potential benefit of vibration to enhance fluid transport, remodeling of inappropriate fibrotic repair after trauma, and optimization of joint range of motion. If done appropriately, rhythmic stretch can recreate correct motion characteristics through controlled plastic deformation by varying the force load for desired effect. This involves working more with the physics of connective tissue than with neurocoordination of tissue tone. Additionally, the psychological effects of rhythmic rocking confirm the natural state of tissue, very much at home with oscillation. The potential for pain relief through rhythmic afferent input, according to the gate theory of pain sensation, is discussed in Chapter 8.

The latter part of this book presents many useful examples of clinical application of rhythmic technique. I think they are well worth reading.

Method Rhythmique d'Harmonization Myotensive

In a hybrid method, growing from a different osteopathic root, Michel Frère describes another approach to rhythmic release. Frère introduces his method in three fashions: historical development, a physiological model, and applied methodology. He cites among influences his experience with Mademoiselle Mezières and her successors Philippe Souchard as well as Godelieve Struyf-Denys. The latter teacher further articulated the concept of "muscle chains" as a basic organizing principle of the body. This influence contributes regional postural patterns of balance against gravity. Frère attributes the implementation of the extremities as long levers, with rhythm and the use of body weight, to John Wernham. Influence by Rolfing methods and the work of Fred Mitchell, Kabatt, Feldenkrais, and Gerda Alexander are also acknowledged.[13]

Principles of the technique include the use of the practitioner's body weight to mobilize the patient and the use of extremity leverage to affect more central aspects of the patient's body. The practitioner's body is grounded as he or she works from a standing position. Frère prefers to work barefoot. The hands work together to both position and push to minimize inappropriate sensory input from tense muscle while monitoring for change in tension. With hands firmly involved, many of the mobilizations occur by the practitioner rocking his or her own body, in firm contact with the patient, on flexed knees to convey the rhythmic force. The source of this harmonizing force is the firm contact of the barefooted practitioner with the earth.

Another idiosyncrasy of the method is a customized table placed at knee height, with side cutouts to allow the practitioner to get closer to the axis of the body.

Treatment is essentially a dialogue between the system of the practitioner and that of the patient. The former adopts an attitude of non-regard, allowing the hands to sense imbalance in the link of the postural chains. The goal of the method[14] is intuitively to reestablish equilibrium within the neuromuscular-skeletal system as well as between this system and the environment. The neuromuscular-skeletal system includes the muscles, their parallel and series connective tissue elements, as well as the articulations.

In health, the primary anti-gravity system of the body is the osseous system. The fascial (aponeurotic) system distributes force and the muscle system accommodates shifts in the center of gravity. The central nervous system integrates the inputs from peripheral proprioceptors to readjust balance. With trauma or strain, maintenance of inappropriate muscle tension, and co-activation of the alpha and gamma motor neurons, the muscular system is allowed to assume the anti-gravity role normally reserved to the skeletal system. This is an inappropriate use of energy and the system becomes strained and symptomatic.

In practice, Method Rhythmique d'Harmonization Myotensive is clearly an oscillatory connective tissue technique. As just mentioned, as a theoretical base for the method, Frère includes a sometimes detailed but often implied description of the balance by the central nervous system between alpha and gamma motor neuron systems modified by golgi tendon innervation. However, beyond reciting this hypothesis proposed by Irwin Korr in 1974, little is added to fill the gap between the intention to normalize and the detailed functional dynamics of the system.[15]

The greater part of this book describes procedures based on my experience; these represent a comprehensive approach to articulation of the points of the spine and extremities. This latter, practical section of Frère's work is extremely valuable as a sharing of ideas for focusing articular force to optimize body mobility. The feature of bodywork as an art form comes forth clearly in his book.

References

[1] Littlejohn, John Martin. "Rhythmicity," unpublished paper distributed at meridianinstitute.com

[2] Wernham, John. *Rhythm in Osteopathy* (Maidstone, England: Institute of Classical Osteopathy, 2003).

[3] Ibid., 28.

[4] Wernham, John, and Christopher Campbell. *The Osteopathic Technique and Philosophy of John Wernham,* video (Maidstone, England: Institute of Classical Osteopathy, 1996).

[5] Lederman, Eyal. *Harmonic Technique* (Edinburgh, Scotland: Churchill Livingston, 2000).

[6] Lederman, Eyal. *Fundamentals of Manual Therapy: Physiology, Neurology and Psychology* (Edinburgh, Scotland: Churchill Livingston, 1997).

[7] Lederman, 2000. Op. cit.

[8] Lederman, 1997. Op. cit., 28.

[9] Lederman, 1997. Op. cit.

[10] Jones, Lawrence. *Jones Strain CounterStrain,* 2nd ed. (Boise: Jones Strain-CounterStrain, Inc, 1995).

[11] Mitchell, Fred. *The Muscle Energy Manual,* vol. 1 (East Lansing, Mich.: MET Press, 1995), 9–11.

[12] Schalow, Giselher, and Y. Blanc. "Electromyographic identification of spinal oscillator patterns and recoupling patterns and recoupling in a patient with incomplete spinal cord lesion: Oscillator formation training as a method of improving motor activities," *Gen. Physiol. Biophys,* 15(1), 1996, 121–220.

[13] Frère, Michel. *Methode Rhythmique d'Harmonization Myotensive* (Charleroi, Belgium: Osteopathic Management Company, SA, 1985), 7–9.

[14] Ibid., 16.

[15] Korr, Irwin. "Research and Practice—A Century Later," A. T. Still Memorial Lecture, *Journal of the American Osteopathic Association,* (73), 1973, 362–370.

Chapter 6

Other Contemporary Uses
of Rhythmic Release

Trager's Moving and Working Softly

Another compatible approach to movement therapy that integrates rhythmic motion is Trager work. Milton Trager intuitively fell in love with motion and the related feelings it precipitated in him. Committed to discovering more and sharing it with others, he pursued a degree in medicine simply to have the license to heal. Empirically, doing gymnastics on the beach with this brother and friends, he appreciated and explored the potential for relaxed, graceful, "easy" motion to build strength and to impart confident and pleasurable feelings. He later made a connection between pain, inappropriately retained emotional stress, and dysfunctional muscle tension patterns.

His methods to release tension tend to be divisible into two venues: autonomous, intentionally guided motion referred to as "Mentastics," and table work. In neither approach is specific technique emphasized; rather, the focus is on the person-to-person transmission or induction of free, easy, and quality motion through receptive tissues to remove blockages. Awareness of quality of motion is the guiding principle. Coaxing, rather than directing or moving tissue, is the vehicle for change. The process begins with the practitioner adopting a relaxed, meditative state and maximizing his or her intuitive sensitivity.[1]

Nonproductive or inefficient postures are often the cause of symptoms. These postures and movements are the result of internalization of stressful experiences. Letting go of inappropriate dysfunctional patterns of posture and movement as induced by these stressors is essential for healing. Trager methods are designed to induce smooth, rounded, sometimes repetitive motions to allow the body to recognize and recall comfortable, functional patterns of motion.

In table work, the beginning point is body contact between patient and practitioner. In a condition of state-dependent learning, the physical and psychologically fluid state of the practitioner is transmitted to the patient. If successful, the patient's body-mind recognizes this state as a natural and comfortable one. "The practitioner loads the atmosphere with the 'virus' of relaxation, peace and flowing movement."[2] The practitioner's body transmits motion, and looks for a response in the tissues of the patient. In table work this will often include rhythmic rocking, sensing the resonance or vibrancy of tissues to set the frequency. Therapeutic effect is achieved by imparting motion, often rhythmic, to patients until they recognize and integrate relaxed soft movements into their own posture, movement habits, and attitude.

> Practitioners feel for the most natural frequency of the part being rhythmically moved, and they move in sync with that frequency, forming a resonant system with the receiver that allows optimal energy transfer.[3]

However, with the technique's emphasis on working spontaneously through feeling, protocols cannot be explicitly described. "The approach is free form and seeks to free the form of the body."[4]

Through his lifetime, Milton Trager spread this love of motion and developed his thoughts and practices into a teachable system called Trager work. He developed a system of personally performed exercises to achieve the same goals. Emphasizing the connection between movement and attitude, he coined the term Mentastics for his routines. Rather than representing an offshoot, Mentastics represents an organized approach to where Trager began in his youth, with experiments in smooth, soft motion. They are therapeutic in their own right but also prepare the practitioner as an effective operator. Trager's teaching methods remained largely empirical and training in this area remains largely limited to licensed workshops.

Vibromuscular Harmonization Technique

Building on the gentle, inductive techniques of Tom Bowen, an inspired self-taught Australian bodyworker, Jock Roddock integrated aspects of intuitive intentionality to a manual protocol known as Vibromuscular Harmonization Technique (VHT). Bowen had recognized, as others have already described, that symptoms and many conditions represent inappropriate body tension patterns. Through fifty years of practice, he developed an approach to creating the opportunity for muscular reeducation to functional, efficient, relaxed posture. Vibration was a minimal component of "the move," as his intervention was described. Basically, the move consisted of identification of location of the problem, then creating, through superficial stretching of the skin, an opportunity for proprioceptive resetting. A greater part was development of the setting, by attention, positive emotions, and gentle contact, in which muscular reeducation could take place, much as the goal of Trager work.

VHT involves the same development of the positive interaction to facilitate change. However, the principle of application of force is altered in intent and method. In Bowen work, the intent is to soothe stressed tissue. VHT's operative principle is to create a chaotic state through stretch and vibration at the point of focal tension, thus creating the opportunity for change. This is accomplished in a two-step process. The move is preceded by a challenge. We begin by drawing lax skin across the edge of a muscle where this focused increase in tension creates a counteracting resistance in the soft tissue that has been suddenly tightened. This move consists of a cross-fiber return movement across the challenged tissue. As a result, the muscle returns in a recoil to its original position and length. This happens suddenly as the tissue returns to its natural resonant frequency.

These maneuvers are executed with fingertip or thumb contact, with coordinated breathing and thought intention.

The method is very different than osteopathic approaches and many other manual approaches in that the judgment of diagnosis is seen as invading the spontaneity of the interaction and the opportunity offered the patient. Though not stated in osteopathic terms, the VHT challenge and move appear to be a dynamic rapid application of indirect followed by direct myofascial release.

References

[1] Liskin, Jack. *Moving Medicine: The Life and Word of Milton Trager, MD* (Barrytown, N.Y.: Station Hill Press, 1996).
[2] Ibid., 131.
[3] Ibid., 136.
[4] Ibid., 133.

Chapter 7

Bioenergetic Models Involving Vibration

Bioenergetics—Poetry and Science

The basic premise of most oscillatory or vibratory therapies is that vibration, or the rhythmic processing of energy, is an essential aspect of matter and therefore of living tissue. The concept is often associated with the relationship in physics regarding the interconvertibility of matter and energy. However, over time the nature of this interrelationship has been expressed in a variety of ways. As scientific applications of these principles have lagged, philosophical, poetic, and spiritual interpretations of this relationship have emerged. Despite the credibility of this intuitive connection with the lay public, such expressions have often alienated the scientific community. Even in this strained climate, however, a steady stream of legitimate scientists have found it natural and necessary to operate in the bioenergetic paradigm.

Neurophysiological Validation

Harold Burr, who inspired Fulford, was a well-published, well-regarded classical neurophysiologist. Curious about the possibility of demonstrating a biological life field, he monitored by voltmeter the galvanic response of trees, from 1938 until 1968. He demonstrated consistency between trees in their response to change of seasons, sunlight and darkness, cycles of the moon, and sunspots. With a medical colleague, Dr. Leonard Ravitz, he surveyed the similar life field of 430 human individuals, and more particularly analyzed the data for diagnostic potential for ovarian cancer.[1]

Inspired by Burr, Robert Becker, MD, an orthopedic surgeon working for the United States Veterans Administration, investigated the properties of this life field.

Becker had revisited many of the same issues and literature in his quest to investigate the body's capacity and mechanisms for healing. His work sheds further light on the electromagnetic aspects of the body.

Initially working out the bioelectric properties of wellness, trauma, and healing in limb regeneration in the salamander model, Becker saw parallels in the healing process in humans, especially in fractures, and in younger children. Limb regeneration and fracture healing involve the reproduction of appropriate materials as well as the restoration of bodily form. He questioned what directed this healing process.[2]

Becker validated the observation that trauma to a limb induced a current of injury, with a positive charge in the limb relative to the trunk, and that in the early stages, there is a conversion to a negative charge. He noted in humans and salamanders that the extremities had a negative baseline while the trunk and head had a positive baseline. He also noted a native DC current that was distributed through the nervous system of an organism; this current was distinct from the AC-like axonal propagation of depolarization of the action potential. The extent and strength of the DC charge could be altered by cutting a nerve, administering anesthesia, or otherwise manipulating the state of consciousness of the organism.

The practical result of his work was the clinical application of electric current to facilitate fracture healing, especially in fractures that did not join correctly in the early stages. However, he was quick to point out that to separate this application from an understanding of the basic electromagnetic character of the body and its function was inappropriate.[3]

Becker's synopsis of the experimental evidence in *The Body Electric*[4] notes that two key issues, often unappreciated in the initiation of healing, are the electromagnetic impetus for the repair and the quality of the regenerative forces. Both are related to the nature of the electromagnetic field, described above. Some of this material has been adequately covered elsewhere in the study of genetic expression, growth factors, and dedifferentiation of mature tissue to pleuripotent cells with subsequent differentiation into the required cell lines for tissue repair.[5] However, the question of the *form* of the organization seemed to Becker to be dependent on some nondepolarizing aspect of neural function. He goes on to hypothesize and test the theory that the distribution of this formative field in the organism appeared to be that of a semiconductor undergoing conduction and rectification, and allow biochemically active electrons to travel freely in the field.[6] Under these conditions the body would function like an ordered crystal. This deviates from, yet complements, the conventional paradigm of biochemical interaction.

Further Measurements of the Energy Field

Valerie Hunt of UCLA is another established PhD neuroscientist who was incidentally intrigued by the question of electromagnetism in living systems. Hunt, originally a skeptic, experienced a career crisis because of her attempts to study the relationship between thoughts, emotions, and the physical body. After being challenged to do so by her students, she began measuring the neuromuscular activity related to variations in emotional states and found that this led to an investigation of auras and altered states of consciousness and their role in healing.

In the course of further experimentation, she was performing EMG (electromyography) on dancers while they were experiencing altered states of consciousness and was confronted with a variety of EMG anomalies at variance with the view of classical neurophysiologists. Furthermore, she found meaningful relationships in the baseline, that part of the signal of lower amplitude usually filtered out as noise. In this millivolt range, she would measure fluctuations that correlated to changes in the auras reported by auric readers. Using NASA's discarded telemetric recording devices and analyzing the power-density and frequency spectrograms, she demonstrated a field that oscillated at frequencies of 250 to above 20,000 Hertz. Further, by manipulating this field in a Mu room, an electromagnetically isolated space, she showed that the field was reactive to changes in the electromagnetic environment and that these changes registered as subjective emotional changes in the patient, including fatigue, stress, and anxiety. Her conclusions were summarized:

> Although composed of the same electrons as inert substances, the human energy field absorbs and throws off energy dynamically. It interacts with and influences other matter whereas fields associated with inert matter react passively. Again, there have been many names associated with this known energy, chi, life force, prana, odic force, and aura.[7]

She drew parallels between the frequency and voltage patterns generated by her data and those chaos attractor functions found in analyses of brain waves, weather data, and other natural phenomena. It would appear that these attractor patterns represent the body's own conductive process and that they had consequences for the individual's health.

However, does this contrast with basic cell theory, the basis for most of biochemical interaction in the body? Hunt would argue, echoing Becker:

> Orthopedist Robert Becker's studies and mine give the most extensive evidence that healing occurs through changes in the electromagnetic field. At the cellular level of molecular circuits, there are endless electro-windings as well as microtubular array of collagen, that is, connective tissue, the support structure of all tissue. At every level through the body, from the cell, to molecule, to atom, there are structural evidences of the intrinsic electromagnetism of life. The whole body oscillates. It has even been speculated that the non-resistive superconductive circuits at the molecular level intimately connect life on a global basis.[8]

She continues:

> Because the human energy field is so resilient, manipulation techniques such as hands-on healing, subtle energy devices, and body therapies introducing subtle energy into the system can more effectively preserve health than those therapies using chemical or mechanical intervention. I believe controlling chaos anywhere in the body via the field will be faster and more enduring than testing specific biological subsystems.
>
> Hands-on and healing by one's presence emphasize the transaction between two people, each with an intent, one to become well and the other to serve as a catalyst. I believe the best healer does not attempt to heal; that belongs to the person desiring to be healed. But rather the healer intends

to present a positive, enlightened presence to manifest a strong, radiant, complete field and encourage the ill field to change.[9]

Hunt cites supporting data regarding integration of physiology, consciousness, and emotional processes. This led her to a career change where she used this research as a basis for biofeedback in individuals with psychological and emotional problems. She now is translating as much of her work as possible into a more easily understandable treatment modality.

Interrelationship of Structure and Function—Tensegrity

In the 1990s Donald Ingber began to mirror Burr in the exploration and expression of a higher level of intracellular and extracellular organization of living tissue, guided by electromagnetic relationships.[10] Ingber began by applying to biological structures the terminology and principles of structural integrity developed by architect-visionary Buckminster Fuller. Fuller used the term *tensegrity* to describe structures whose stability, or tensional integrity, depended on the dynamic balance between discontinuous compression elements connected by continuous-tension cables.[11]

Ingber's major argument reflected Burr's criticism of cellular biology in which study was done under the presumption that cellular contents could adequately be described as an organized nucleus and organelles floating in a suspension of homogenous protoplasm.

As cellular biology and observational methods had progressed, Ingber attested to the functional significance of a higher level of order within the cell. In later work,[12] he avoided altogether the language of analogy to a tensegrity model and simply described the functional significance of the tiered orders of structural organization that exist even to the molecular intracellular level. This structural continuum of the gross connective tissue matrix of the extracellular milieu extends to finer levels of organization, to include extracellular and intercellular integrins, the cell membrane, and actinomysin intercellular microtubules. The functional significance is captured in the following quotes.

> Our bodies are complex hierarchical structures, and hence mechanical deformation of whole tissues results in coordinated structural rearrangements on many different size scales.[13]
>
> In fact, cell-generated tensional forces appear to play a central role in the development of virtually all living tissues and organs even in neural tissue, such as the retina and brain.[14]

Ingber sees the significance of this as complementary to genetically initiated transduction of proteins. In this appreciation of the role of mechanotransduction, as he uses the term, he gives numerous examples of specific cells reacting to subtle shear forces that initiate alteration in size, shape, and function through the expression of proteins in response to the stress.[15]

Crossover to Quantum Physics as It Relates to Tissue

Mae-wan Ho, after an extensive, lifelong journey through biochemistry, genetics, evolutionary biology, and quantum physics, adds another layer to this theme of electromolecular wholism which is the body.[16] She, like Burr and Becker, is sharply critical of the historic study of cell function by homogenation and fractional analysis of cell contents. Using the continuous connectivity of structure described by Ingber and others, she makes the case for an extension of the electron exchange process in classical metabolic pathways as a general principle of cell, and organism, function. She extends this complexity to describe the continuum of organization from the gross to the molecular level where electromagnetic interaction is most clearly recognized. She hypothesizes, cogently, that cellular connectivity already serves as a network, describing it thus:

> ...organized flow of electric currents—meticulously coordinated from the very short range of intermolecular charge transfers right up through many intermediate levels of space and time to currents traversing the whole organism—constitutes what I have referred elsewhere to as the coherent electrodynamic field that underlies living organization.[17]

Consider in this context again the quote from A. T. Still: "The fascia proves itself to be the matrix of life and death."[18]

Beyond hydrogen bonding and the phosphorylation-dephosphorylation of adenosine diphosphate, electrons are free-flowing, as in a crystal lattice, within the context of this electromolecular body complex. In other words, the body tissues function as semiconductors in certain closely controlled metabolic conditions, yet to be properly understood. Phase coherence and changes of phase state are more likely to define the time scale of physiological events than conventional Newtonian convection.[19]

Coherence and changes of phase state are aspects of neuroscience explored in the Chapter 8 discussion of neurophysiology of muscle spasm and relaxation underlying the theory of effectiveness of Facilitated Oscillatory Release.

Intentionality and Psychobiology

Once the reality of electromagnetic regulation on the scale of mass effect is accepted, the means of modifying phase states needs to be discussed. Many of the manual methods describe the importance of the mental state, attention, or intention of the practitioner. Can thoughts change bioregulatory parameters?

Jacqueline Bousquet,[20] a PhD in biology having done research in endocrinology and immunology, builds on many of the influences of Ho, but expresses the compatible integrity of quantum bioscience, psychology, and theology, especially when interpreted in a gnostic-esoteric sense. In this context, the interconvertibility of matter and energy in the atomic-subatomic and molecular level is appreciated as the basis of matter, of life, and of emotional and spiritual interaction. As proclaimed elsewhere and through history, the universe is a seamless whole and this is consistent with, not contradictory to, science if completely understood.[21]

In the venue of our current interest, Bousquet underscores that energetic resonance of atoms, molecules, organs, and individuals, and that changing the level of vibration creates change in structure and function.[22] Further, she cites:

Forme = Energie = Information = Temps [*Temps* translates as time][23]

In this context, the vibrational information required for life is stored in energetic bonds and the long axis of DNA.[24] To simplify, Bousquet proposes that a change of heart, a spiritual rebirth, reflects a conformational, informational change even to the cellular level, and can be mediated by the parameters of spiritual interaction, including mind.

Proteomics—After Sequencing Human DNA

Under the title of psychobiology, in a more contemporary expression, Ernest Rossi resonates with all these ideas and develops a model, intended to validate psychotherapy, in which social and environmental stimuli are described as affecting neural circuits. However, Rossi goes beyond the description of neuroreceptor chemistry into a new expression of genetics, the field now known as protein genomics, or proteomics. This area of study is involved with exploring the coordinated expression or production of proteins in the organized function of the organism.

Rossi cites numerous investigators working with clock genes and immediate early genes, demonstrating that interactions with the environment can alter the transcription of proteins and alter behavior in rapid fashion. He proposes these mechanisms as responsible for learning, mood states, and consciousness itself. Although Rossi's descriptions are intended to underpin the process of psychotherapy, they show promise regarding many psychosomatic conditions, including pain states. As such, the dynamics suggest a further scientifically valid role for "anti-stress" maneuvers through a variety of physical, verbal, and nonverbal inputs from a practitioner.

Nicholas Handoll, a British DO with a grounding in cranial osteopathy, reinterprets the principles and observations of William Sutherland in terms of quantum mechanics, after being so encouraged by Rollin Becker, Sutherland's student. Handoll outlines the basic hierarchy of matter, including our tissues, in this quantum physics perspective and associates the experiential contact with "the Potency" as the engagement of two individuals, patient and practitioner, on a level beyond that of common sense, or biomechanics, yet none the less real.[25]

Water Memory

Complementing this analysis of bioelectric effects is the further consideration of the role of water in biological function and information storage. Ho, Burr, and Bousquet all include the role of water molecules and the interaction of hydrogen bonds, which lend electrons to many processes, as a key feature of the energetic process of the body.

Masuru Emoto[26] has proposed that water itself, possibly through change of quantum phase states, has the capacity to store the energy communicated in thought and intention. In a semi-repeatable method, Emoto has developed a protocol for analysis of the qualities of ice crystals from water that has been "charged" with thoughts. Crystals made from water imparted with negative thoughts or emotions yield asymmetric, distorted, or amorphous crystal forms. Crystals from positively charged water demonstrate symmetry, delicacy, and aesthetically pleasant shapes.

This work, thus far, shows scientific limitations in its qualitative nature and variability with replication. However, this may be perceived as a developing frontier as much as a blind alley. Interest in Japanese culture in this area of exploration and expression is high, partly because of a traditional role for vibration, thought, and energy in acupuncture and in the nature of Zen and other Buddhist practices that deal with the regulation or mastery of consciousness.

Reviews of this same area of interest are also found in James Oschman's *Energy Medicine* and *Energy Medicine in Therapeutics and Human Performance*,[27,28] as well as Richard Gerber's *Vibrational Medicine*.[29]

Awareness of the clinical relevance of vibration is the foundation of much of Eastern medicine. Cosmic harmonies in the five-element tradition of Chinese medicine, chi gong, the yin and yang of Buddhist cosmology expressed in various forms, as well the particular implementations of acupuncture all rely on the reality of vibration at various frequency ranges. More recently, the new expression of the Japanese concept of *hado,* wave or vibration, has surfaced in healing work. Although the particulars of some of these expressions are relevant in their sense of consilience, particulars in clinical application will be dealt with in a separate book.

References

[1] Burr, Harold. *Blueprint for Immortality: The Electric Patterns of Life* (Essex, England: Saxton Walden, 1972).

[2] Becker, Rollin. *The Body Electric: Electromagnatism and the Foundation of Life* (New York: William Morrow, 1985), 5.

[3] Ibid., 98.

[4] Ibid., 95–102.

[5] Ibid., 55.

[6] Ibid., 93–99.

[7] Hunt, Valerie. *Infinite Mind: Science of the Human Vibration of Consciousness* (Malibu, Calif.: Malibu Publishing Co., 1989), 20.

[8] Ibid., 240.

[9] Ibid., 265.

[10] Ingber, Donald. "The riddle of morphogenesis: A question of solution chemistry or molecular cell engineering?" *Cell,* (75), 1993, 1249–1252.

[11] Fuller, Buckminster. *Synergetics* (New York: Macmillan, 1975).

[12] Ingber, Donald. "Mechanobiology and diseases of mechanotransduction," *Annals of Medicine,* 35(8), 2003, 5645–5677.

[13] Ibid., 5646.

[14] Ibid., 5648.

[15] Ibid.

[16] Ho, Mae-wan. *The Rainbow and the Worm: The Physics of Organisms* (Singapore: World Scientific Publishing Co., 1998).

[17] Ibid., 132

[18] Still, Andrew. *Philosophy of Osteopathy* (Indianapolis: American Academy of Osteopathy; 1977), 89. Originally self-published in Kirksville, Mo., in 1899.

[19] Ho. Op. cit., 113.

[20] Bousquet, Jacqueline. *Au Coeur du Vivant* (St. Michel du Bologne, France: St. Michel Editions, 1992).

[21] Ibid., 154.

[22] Ibid., 155.

[23] Ibid.

[24] Ibid., 156.

[25] Handoll, Nicholas. *Anatomy of Potency* (Hereford, England: Osteopathic Supply Ltd, 2000).

[26] Emoto, Masaru. *Messages from Water* (Tokyo: Kyoikusha, Hado.net, 2001).

[27] Oschman, James. *Energy Medicine: The Scientific Basis* (Edinburgh, Scotland: Churchill Livingston; 2000).

[28] Oschman, James. *Energy Medicine in Therapeutics and Human Performance* (Boston: Elsevier Science, 2003).

[29] Gerber, Richard. *Vibrational Medicine: New Choices for Healing Ourselves* (Sante Fe, N.M.: Bear and Co., 1988).

Part II

Principles and Support for Facilitated Oscillatory Release

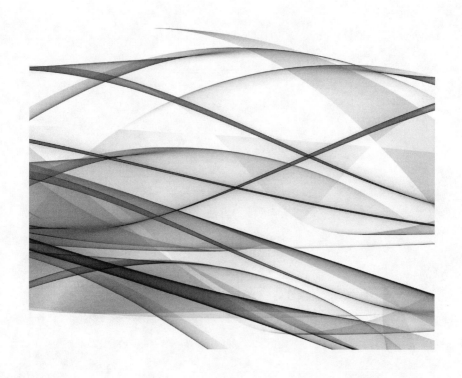

Chapter 8

Physiological Basis for Rhythmic Diagnosis and Treatment, and Effectiveness of Oscillatory Force

Facilitated Oscillatory Release—Supportive Science

Facilitated Oscillatory Release (FOR) is quite compatible with concepts and explanations described in the preceding chapters. However, while a wholistic, solidly grounded scientific validation still lags behind, the reason for effectiveness is presented here in terms of advanced neurophysiological theory, complemented by classical principles of connective tissue work.

Coordination of Motion

Osteopaths and many other bodyworkers have long held that health is defined by the capacity for unimpeded motion and that the body has self-regulatory capacity. The extent and implications of this internal synergy is progressively elucidated as bioscientific knowledge advances. Similarly, many of Still's other particularly intuitive insights into the integral functions of the vascular, lymphatic, and nervous systems have been validated by later scientific discoveries.

Most models of osteopathic diagnosis and treatment pay attention to local restriction or regional articular synergy and coordination in motion patterns.[1] Others pay attention to concurrent muscle hyperemia and neural facilitation,[2,3] while still others correlate segmental articular restriction with reciprocally impaired visceral function. Several models of osteopathic diagnosis and treatment have enlarged the scope to consider the whole person. One of these, the connective tissue approach, has evolved apparently out of osteopathy in the cranial field as an appreciation of the properties and behavior of the fascial system.[4] Additionally, the particular expression of William Johnston, DO, on functional technique stresses diagnosis and treatment to optimize the function of mobile segments in a mobile system.[5]

Johnston's phenomenological approach acknowledges the theoretical operation of a central pattern regulator as part of the self-regulating mobile system, but treats it as a "black box," without correlation with more recent neuroscience. Robert Fulford, DO, added an appreciation of the fascia as the circuitry in a bioelectric system responding to trauma or nurturance. Fulford's model pricks our intuitive conscience to look more broadly but leans more heavily on the literature readily available to him, largely philosophical and anthropological, with several scientists cited.[6]

Edward Stiles, DO, integrates the idea of tensegrity, a model of interdependence of parts, as a means of expressing the structural interrelatedness of human function.[7] The tensegrity model is helpful in recognizing the complex structural interrelationships within and among regions as well as on different levels of scale in observation. This interrelatedness exists on the nuclear, intracellular, intercellular, and expanded tissue level.

Osteopathic philosophy has always highlighted the crucial interrelationship of structure and function. Progressively, first in relationship to neuroanatomy and then in the connective tissue context, subtle coordinative functional features are being defined and await clinical application.

Neuroreflexive Models

A significant amount of work toward understanding the neu-rofunctional relationships underlying somatic dysfunction has centered on an understanding of reflexes and learning within the peripheral and central nervous systems. One major line of thought began with a hypothesis proposed by Irwin Korr, on the relevance of the gamma motor system. Korr's hypothesis was that the experience of dysfunction is due to the mis-coordination of the neural circuit (gamma afferent and alpha and gamma motor neuron response) that coordinates the resting length of a muscle. After strain, this mis-coordination would cause the muscle to remain in a semi-contracted state, which could cause postural imbalance or muscle pain.[8] In other words, proprioceptive mis-coordination is primary and the nerve conduction of pain signals as well as articular asymmetries are secondary.

A competitive hypothesis for the cause of the segmental dys-function was summarized by Richard VanBuskirk,[9] proposing that nociceptive rather than the proprioceptive afferent input was the primary cause of persistent muscle hypertonia and spinal facilita-tion. This theme is reiterated with a high degree of sophistication by Frank Willard, PhD,[10] who cites the research of Anderson and Winterson.[11] Anderson and Winterson infer neural coordination at the cord and brain levels to be driven by nociception or pain sensation. Pain then would be the primary cause of the muscle contraction, rather than the effect.

Anderson and Winterson's investigations work with spinal fixation in a rat model, involving irritation of a limb resulting in flexion contraction that persists for hours to weeks after spinal cord transection above the segment responsible for the reflex contraction. Although duration of contraction between spinalized and unspinalized rats was the same, force of contraction was significantly greater in spinalized rats, otherwise untreated. N-methyl-D-aspartate (NMDA) had been demonstrated to be a neurotransmitter involved in many excitatory synapses. To demonstrate the role of c-fiber afferent activation in persistence of flexion contractures, a subset of rats was first pretreated with an NMDA antagonist, which resulted in a decrease in strength of contraction in both the spinalized and intact rats.

To further demonstrate c-fiber afferent specificity, a c-fiber neurotoxin, capsaicin, was injected and showed a decrease in force of contraction. Additional structural manipulations included dorsal rhizotomy and removal of the skin of the contracted hind limb. Each maneuver resulted in less of a flexion response, but some flexion persisted until removal of the spine and spinal cord from T13 to L6.

Willard cites the maintenance of some flexion contracture after cutting the dorsal root as proof that contracture persists after interrupting the gamma afferent, alpha efferent loop. He deduces that the pain pathway then is responsible for the persistence of reflex motor response.

In an expanded model, Willard relies on the literature on central sensitization to explain the persistence of chronic pain after the completion of healing of tissue after strain or trauma.[12,13]

Previous Classical Work

Previous work by Steinmetz and Patterson, compatible with Anderson's and Winterson's work, had used the spinal fixation model to demonstrate the importance of spinal and cortical input into peripheral muscle contraction. Their work also showed persistence of flexion until spinal cord transection and they conclude that this demonstrates the influence of dynamic spinal and CNS influences on peripheral reflexes.[14,15]

Early in his work, Patterson proposed a spinal regulatory or facilitated segment model for the explanation of somatic dysfunction, with the following comment:

> In postulating a role for habituation, sensitization, and conditioning in protecting against, producing and maintaining segmental facilitation, I have altered the concept of the role of the spinal neural paths from that of passive transmitters to that of active, vital participation in the mechanism of health and disease.[16]

The progressive weakening of the response in Anderson's and Winterson's experiment after successive interventions suggests the complementarity of numerous influences at a variety of anatomical sites within the reflex pathways of a facilitated spinal segment. It demonstrates only that the spinal cord is a necessary part of this regulatory apparatus. The study does legitimately challenge the simplicity of the gamma reflex loop hypothesis.

> A bilateral (dorsal) rhizotomy which assuredly severs Ia muscle spindles afferents did not affect persistent flexion. This argues for an asymmetric, hyper excitability in neurons that are in *premotor circuits* [italics added] and not enhancements of Ia afferent drives to motor neurons.[17]

However, cutting the dorsal root, which eliminates recurrent input to the gamma loop, seems to me to involve also interrupting persistent c-afferent input to the cord. This leaves us with the same challenge presented by Willard to the gamma loop advocates.

One way out of this dilemma is to consider as separate the functions of initiating and maintaining a contraction. The role of neural circuits may be different in each instance.

The classical reflex pathways may be one way of initiating a contraction. Maintenance of such a flexion contracture may require persistence of the initiating pathway. However, more interesting to me is the possible input from peripheral sources (joint pain receptors, postural generators, gamma afferents, stretch receptors) in maintaining a contracture, since it is from the periphery that the osteopathic physician can apply force to intervene in regulatory mechanisms.

Additionally, in this context, the persistence of a previously initiated muscle contraction (reinitiated state) may not need continuous input to be maintained. Rather, it may persist until interrupted by the initiation of a subsequent event. In this instance, in Anderson's and Winterson's experimental model, the muscle has simply been isolated from further potential spinal input. A similar hypothesis for sustained hypertonia has been proposed for the mechanism of muscle fatigue.[18] In this hypothesis, relaxation is dependent on the input of new energy in the form of ATP (adenosine triphosphate), the source of energy in most normal muscle contraction.

In all three of these research models, maintenance of the pain and muscle tension rely on altered reflex circuits. Actual muscle activity is conceptualized as dependent on continual input of some sort. A steady state of dysfunctional hypertonia may have another explanation, as we will now explore.

Another Input—Dynamic Interpretation of Postural Coordination

The preoccupation in the above-cited models is the primacy of the altered reflex pathway in somatic dysfunction. Alterations in the characteristics of the pathways are presumed to be responsible for alterations in function. Many of the clinically observed features of dysfunction and results of manipulative work do not seem to fit with this reflexive model and its emphasis on discrete pathways in which the elements connect or do not connect.

Criticism of the gamma gain hypothesis seems legitimate. But the frequent presence of hypertonic muscle, not initially painful to the patient until firmly pressed by the examiner, points beyond the nociceptive model. Additionally, the remediation of many pain presentations, even chronic, when the correct maneuver is applied disfavors an explanation based on neurochemical modification of thresholds of sensitivity or genetic expression in the central nervous system. Change in the coordinative system and the perception of pain and discomfort are notably more plastic, even in short time courses, than these models seem to allow. To address these points, much of what has been learned about the dynamic features of the neurocoordinative process—binding and coding, phasic resonance, phase coherence patterns, and resonant cell assembly function—seem relevant.

What do I mean by *coding* and *phase coherence patterns*? These terms introduce us to another functional side of neurology beyond the popular model of the final common pathway in muscle activation and reflexive coordination. The anatomical specificity of pathways supporting these previously described hypotheses are indeed essential but represent just a portion of what is occurring in proprioceptive function and maintenance of muscle tone. At one point these anatomical descriptions represented the frontier of knowledge about the nervous system. In this context, these previous models tend to favor the importance of structural relationships in determining function. What follows is intended to be an expansion of our understanding of the pertinent anatomy, the structure, by expanding our appreciation of certain aspects of function relevant to pain and dysfunction.

This further appreciation of the functional aspect of motor activation and the response to stress comes from an area of neurophysiology involved with the specificity in coding and binding in the central nervous system (the way in which sensory stimuli are discriminated, stored, and directed toward response events).

Neuronal population coding has challenged or replaced modular and line-labeled coordination in much of the neurophysiological literature.[19,20,21]

For those yet unfamiliar with this area of study, the analogy between computer hardware and software seems appropriate in comparing the two approaches—they are complementary yet both essential. One era, stressing the importance of connectivity of the depolarization pathways, is giving birth to a newer approach that stresses the temporal relationship between depolarization patterns on these same pathways.

To put this second approach in historical perspective, as early as 1802, working with the problem of color vision, Young challenged the concept of line labeling of specific receptor cells, interconnecting neurons and brain cells dedicated to the sensation of a particular experience. The economy of space in the retina and brain would not accommodate dedicated structures for the range of frequencies perceptible. He proposed the trichromic theory of color vision, including the idea of information coding by receptors.[22] Donald Hebb in the 1940s further elucidated this functional approach to neural coding by proposing that neurons fire as coordinative groups (resonant cell assemblies) and could act concurrently in the transmission of information reflecting different experiences.[23] In Hebb's model, information was transmitted over distance by merging assemblies called *sync fire chains*. Additionally cells underwent post-synaptic changes as part of learning or memory (neural plasticity). The patterns of depolarization, rather than exclusively the locus or synaptic pathway, began to emerge as significant in stimulus recognition. Hebb's language of resonant depolarization of groups of cells (cell assemblies), oscillatory depolarization (resonance), and the persistence of the coherence phase synchrony of these patterns (coherence patterns) and rhythmic dissemination of a potential (sync fire chain) began for many researchers to replace the language of synapse, depolarization, common pathway, and recruitment in describing an event in the CNS—a stimulus recognition, a memory, an association.[24,25,26]

Over time, numerous research scientists followed this lead in viewing this issue of neural coordination, throughout the nervous system, as a coding problem. The total solution is under continuous debate. Some observers highlight certain characteristics of function in the form of the signal traffic on these pathways.[27] The common feature of these theories of coding and binding in the central nervous system is that the organization of activity depends on more than the hardwiring, receptor specificity, and neurotransmitters. Beginning with studies in the brain and retina, it has become apparent that neurons eligible for recruitment in response to stimulation cooperate in depolarization events by firing repetitively, until the stimulus is removed, dominated by another, or extinguished by some other means. This is particularly true of what is termed long-term depolarization. Moreover, the cells participate in groups of cooperatively firing neurons, which cyclically activate one another as a local event (resonant cell assembly), or as a linear event passing the stimulus to another more distant part of the neural system (sync fire chain). Certain nuclei of cells may coordinate the larger pattern of resonant depolarization (neural pattern generators). In this way, this functional redefinition of the nervous system emphasizes the feature of functional resonant coordination, over and above the study of the distribution of pathways, the characteristics of synapses and other cell receptors, and neurotransmitters. The activity is rhythmic, and therefore relevant to our discussion.

The classical osteopathic and chiropractic point of view pay much attention to the spine and spinal nerves. It is worth noting that others have seen this aspect of neural function also in the peripheral nervous system. Beginning in the spinal cord and its peripheral distribution, the body records pain and responses with muscle contraction, or hypertonia, not simply with the continual discharge of a synaptic pathway, but through the pattern of cyclic depolarization within a population of cells (cell assembly). Coordinated activity demonstrates patterns of harmonic resonance, or depolarizations in phase, between nerve or muscle fibers. The relationship of phase coincidence and variation, or coherence, provides a code by which the body regulates activity. The threshold for activation of a function is dependent on coherence or resonance of cells linearly related in a chain (sync fire chain) as the means of communication. The strength of an action potential and its ability to propagate through the network depends on the coordinated phase synchrony of its contributing neurons.

Using microneurographic technology, Windhorst has demonstrated patterns of synchronous firing within groups of neurons involved in a common task (coherence patterns).[28,29]

Furthermore, Zedka[30] and then Farmer[31] have demonstrated that voluntary motion in the periphery involves a pattern of oscillatory micro tremors, in phase with a similar pattern of neuronal depolarization in the spinal cord. The entire neuromuscular coordinative system involves rhythmic function. Curiously, Staude et al.[32] demonstrate that rhythmic voluntary motion affects the initiation of a discrete voluntary motion task.

Phase synchrony or total coherence is equivalent in auditory experience to sounds being of the same pitch. In our sensual experience of hearing, sounds slightly off pitch generate a beat frequency between the two notes. Sounds too far off pitch are perceived as noise, with no harmonic relationship to the original sound. Sounds at resonant intervals, at an octave above or below, again have a harmonic relationship to the first sound. What is proposed in the newer view of resonant cell assembly interaction in the nervous system is that oscillatory depolarization generated in response to a stimulus dominates neural function until one of disharmonic character arises to "swamp" the original pattern and perhaps initiate a new one. Any circuit, including the alpha-gamma system and their afferents, may maintain a depolarization pattern until induced by new inputs to change that pattern.[33]

If such is the case, the coordinative system ought to be able to be influenced by rhythmic afferent input even if externally induced. Such is the case in the work of Swiss physiatrist Giselher Schalow. In an exciting pattern of life work in rehabilitative medicine, working with a population of young patients suffering from partial spinal cord transections, Schalow monitored the phase coordination patterns of depolarization in individual and paired homologous motor neurons in opposite lower extremities and noted different phase relationships in normal and cord-damaged subjects. His aim was to help reestablish more normal neurologic control of the urinary bladder and legs. After application of a repetitive oscillatory input to the distal extremity (patient supported by a harness and bouncing on a spring board), the subjects showed progressive normalization pattern of firing (measured microneurographically) in oscillatory phase between the neurons reapproximating normal functional pattern, and this coincided with progressive return of motor control and independent gait in some subjects.[34,35] In other words, externally applied plus internally initiated rhythmic motion overcame reflexive muscle spasticity that had been preventing normal motion.

Most of our somatic dysfunction does not represent the same extreme case, but I believe the principles apply.

Tonic Vibratory Reflex

In a separate line of scientific investigation, neurophysiologists have observed a phenomenon they call the *tonic vibratory reflex*. Its relevance will be more apparent as we proceed. Long known in the field of muscle physiology, just as were the Hoffman or H-reflex and the stretch reflex, tonic vibratory reflex has awaited a clinical application. It can be described this way. When a vibratory stimulus is applied to muscle, several results occur. Typically, in the blindfolded individual, when an arm muscle belly is vibrated at the appropriate frequency (40–100 Hz), the subject loses a sense of where the limb is in space, and the muscle or its antagonist muscle contracts in an involuntary way. This may be accompanied by an illusory sense of motion, often in the absence of displacement, or spontaneous drift in an intentionally stable arm.[36,37,38,39]

Microneurographic measurement, including in the gamma motor system, correlated with this gross motor activity in the presence of vibration.[40,41,42] Interestingly, the frequency range of applied vibration to initiate this phenomenon corresponds to that used with Dr. Fulford's percussion vibration technique with a frequency range up to 65 Hz. This body of work is consistent with oscillatory depolarization of associated neuromuscular tracks in phase coherence patterns.

Investigation into the particulars of neural coordination is vast; the summary here does not even touch the spectrum of theories. But this discussion highlights the theme of the nervous system as a milieu of dynamic, cyclic processes. More notably, so far, this view of neural coordination has had limited clinical application.[43,44] The concepts and research, however, are key to understanding the neurophysiological underpinnings of FOR.

Connective Tissue Distensibility

Connective tissues, including fascias, are affected by rhythmic motion. Collectively, connective tissue gives form and support to the body. Organs, vessels, nerves, muscles, and bones all share a fibrin matrix, which, combined with other elements, defines the stability and movement characteristics of each anatomical element. Bone incorporates calcium phosphate to lend rigidity and stability to the body. Muscle adds neuroresponsive proteins that enable it to be able to change shape, to adapt and move. But all connective tissue shares a common mesodermal embryologic origin and is replenished after injury by reproliferation of fibrocytes. Striated muscle, a tissue that is distensible on demand, also is derived from this same mesoderm.[45]

The permeating and investing connective tissue of the body is generically called fascia. The fascias have a high fibrin content that is arrayed along the local axis of motion. In some locations it has been given specific names. However, the fascias of the body are a continuous system anatomically, giving credence to the tensegrity model of function described in Chapter 7. The fascias define form, create compartments to separate incompatible chemical processes and to create pressure gradients to aid in transport, and participate in the regional coordination of motion.

Loose connective tissue is a matrix of fibrin, collagen, and amorphous grounds substance. Each element contributes to the strength, resilience, and compliance of connective tissue in its native state. Each defines characteristics of connective tissue in healing from injury. In general terms the elastin serves to allow controlled, reversible deformation under strain. Fibrin serves as a check on the extent of this compliance much as do the fibrin filaments of ligaments in muscle. The ground substance serves as a conduit for nutrients and waste products as well as a medium for cytoactive elements.

These connective tissues are living tissue and as such have a certain ability to respond to changes in the environment. In areas in which greater force is regularly encountered, connective tissue further modifies its conformation, becoming linear in its fibrous orientation in ligaments and tendons, and more densely packed and calcified in tubercles and bones. Extreme stress in bone leads to remodeling, osteoarthritic changes, and osteophyte formation. Yet, even bone in the living mammal is a vascular, pink, pliable material that is responsive and serves many vital functions. It is far from the isolated dry, white, brittle specimen.

Strain on linear connective tissue also results, as we have said, in stress and possibly deformation. A certain amount of such distortion is physiologically necessary as part of the low-pressure circulatory aspects of the system. However, isolated excessive strain as well as sudden forces, as in traumatic impacts, may cause deformation beyond the elastic limit of the tissues. This may result in a semi-permanent distortion of the connective tissue matrix, notably the alteration of fibrin bonds. This is the area of most interest in manipulative therapy in which reintroduction of force creates the occasion for the resolution of the results of strain. The relative permanence of this deformation is due to the exothermic nature of the chemical reactions involved. In other words, in trauma or strain, energy is absorbed and released with a net loss. Technically, the phenomenon is called *hysteresis;* in some contexts this is termed the energy of injury.[46,47]

Further strain transmitted beyond the degree that can be absorbed by the loose and fascial connective tissue matrix may be absorbed by the muscular, ligamentous, articular cartilaginous or bony elements of the musculoskeletal system, besides organs.

Return to normal form and function is possible only with the reintroduction of energy appropriate and sufficient to reverse the process. Such force must be directional and localized so as to recreate the correct conformation of the tissue in question.

Classically, several forms of manipulation have been used as catalysts to allow the injured and deformed tissues to find a conformation similar to their pre-injury state. The presumption, which seems empirically verified, is that this reduces pain and restores normal function.

References

[1] Fryette, Harrison. *Principles of Osteopathic Technique* (Kirksville, Mo.: Journal Printing Company, 1994).

[2] Ward, Robert, ed. *Foundations for Osteopathic Medicine,* 2nd ed. (Philadelphia: Lippincott Williams and Wilkins, 2003), 137.

[3] Jones, Lawrence. *Jones Strain CounterStrain,* 2nd ed. (Boise: Jones Strain-CounterStrain Inc., 1995), 13–15.

[4] Sutherland, William. *Teachings in the Science of Osteopathy,* Anne Wales, ed. (Dallas: Sutherland Cranial Teaching Foundation, 1990), 278ff.

[5] Johnston, William, and Harry Friedman. *Functional Methods: A Manual for Palpatory Skill Development in Osteopathic Examination and Manipulation of Motor Function* (Indianapolis: American Academy of Osteopathy, 1995).

[6] Comeaux, Zachary. *Robert Fulford, DO, and the Philosopher Physician* (Seattle: Eastland Press, 2002).

[7] Stiles, Edward. "Osteopathy: The clinical approach of a complex thinker, A. T. Still, MD," paper delivered at Convocation of the American Academy of Osteopathy, Colorado Springs, 2001.

[8] Korr, Irwin. "Proprioceptors and somatic dysfunction," *Journal of the American Osteopathic Association,* (74), 1975, 646.

[9] VanBuskirk, Richard. "Nociceptive Reflex and Somatic Dysfunction: A Model," *Journal of the American Osteopathic Association,* 90(9), 1990, 792ff.

[10] Willard, Frank. "The Nociceptive Model of Somatic Dysfunction in the Peripheral Nervous System," presentation to West Virginia School of Osteopathic Medicine, Nov. 2002.

[11] Anderson, M., and B. Winterson. "Properties of peripherally induced persistent hind limb flexion in rest: Involvement of N–methyl-D-aspartate receptors and capsaicin-sensitive afferents," *Brain Research*, (678), 1995, 140–150.

[12] Willard, Frank. "Anatomy and Osteopathic Medicine," lecture on videotape, Convocation of American Academy of Osteopathy, Ontario, Calif. (Indianapolis: American Osteopathic Association, 2003).

[13] Willard, Frank. "The influence of somatic dysfunction (nociceptive model) on rheumatological diseases," lecture on videotape, Convocation of American Academy of Osteopathy, Colorado Springs (Indianapolis: American Osteopathic Association, 2004).

[14] Steinmetz, Joseph, and Michael Patterson. "Central and Peripheral Influences on Retention of Postural Asymmetry in Rats," *Journal of Comparative and Physiological Psychology*, 96(1), 1982, 4–11.

[15] Steinmetz, Joseph, Michael Patterson, and David Molea. "Long-term retention of a peripherally induced flexor reflex alteration in rats," *Brain Research*, (327), 1985, 312–315.

[16] Patterson, Michael. "A model mechanism for spinal segmental facilitation," *Yearbook* (Indianapolis: American Academy of Osteopathy, 1976), 17–24.

[17] Anderson, M., and B. Winterson, 1995. Op. cit.

[18] McComas, Alan. *Skeletal Muscle: Form and Function* (Champaign, Ill.: Human Kinetics, 1996).

[19] Sakurai, Y. "How do cell assemblies encode information in the brain?" *Neurosci Biobehav Rev*, 23(6), 1999, 785–796.

[20] Sanger, T. D. "Neural population codes," *Curr Opin Neurobiol*, 13(2), 2003, 238–249.

[21] Doetsch, G. S. "Patterns in the brain: Neuronal population coding in the somatosensory system," *Physiol Behav*, 69(1–2), 2000, 187–201.

[22] Erickson, R. "The evolution and implications of population and modular neural coding ideas," *Prog Brain Res*, (130), 2001, 9–29.

[23] Spatz, H-C. "Hebb's concept of synaptic plasticity and neuronal cell assemblies," *Behavioral Brain Research*, (78), 1996, 3–7.

24 Farmer, S. "Rhythmicity, synchronization and binding in human and primate motor systems," *J Physiol,* 509(1), 1998, 3–14.

25 Sakurai, Y. "Population coding by cell assemblies—what really is in the brain," *Neuroscience Res,* 26(1), 1996, 1625.

26 Valera, F. "Resonant cell Assemblies: A new approach to cognitive functions and neuronal synchrony," *Biol Res,* (28), 1995, 81–95.

27 Spatz, H-C. Op. cit.

28 Windhorst, Uwe. *How Brain Like Is the Spinal Cord? Interacting Cell Assemblies in the Nervous System* (New York: Springer Verlag, 1988).

29 Windhorst, Uwe. "The Spinal Cord and Its Brain: Representations and models: To what extent do forebrain mechanisms appear at brainstem spinal cord levels," *Progress in Neurobiology;* (49), 1996, 381–414.

30 Zedka, M. "Phasic activity in the human erector spinae during repetitive hand motions," *J Physiol,* 504(3), 1997, 727–734.

31 Farmer, S. Op. cit.

32 Staude, G., R. Dengler, and W. Wolf. "The discontinuous nature of motor execution in merging discrete and rhythmic movements in a single joint system: The phase entrainment effect," *Biol Cybe,* 86(6), 2002, 427–443.

33 Zedka, M. Op. cit.

34 Schalow, Giselher. "Spinal oscillators in man under normal and pathological conditions," *Electromyog Clin Neurophysio,* (33), 1993, 409–426.

35 Schalow, Giselher, and G. Zach. "Neuronal Reorganization through Oscillator Formation Training in Patients with CNS Lesions," *J Peripheral Nervous System,* (3), 1993, 165–188.

36 Roll, J. P., and J. C. Gilhodes. "Proprioceptive sensory codes mediating movement trajectory perception: Human hand vibration-induced drawing illusions," *Can J Physiol Pharmacol,* (73), 1995, 295–304.

37 Gilhodes, J. C., V. S. Gurfinkle, and J. P. Roll. "Role of Ia muscle spindle afferents in post-contraction and post-vibration motor effect genesis," *Neuroscience Letters,* (135), 1992, 247–251.

38 Burke, D., and K. E. Hagnbarth. "The responses of human muscle spindle endings to vibration during isometric contraction," *J Physiol,* (261), 1976, 695–711.

[39] Prochazka, A., and P. St. J. Trend. "Instability in human forearm movement studied with feed-back-controlled muscle vibration," *J Physiol,* (402), 1988, 421–442.

[40] Martin, B., and H. Park. "Analysis of the tonic vibratory reflex: Influence of vibration variables on motor unit synchrony and fatigue," *Eur J Appl Physiol,* (75), 1997, 504–511.

[41] Roll, J. P., and J. C. Gilhodes. Op. cit.

[42] Gilhodes, J. C., V. S. Gurfinckle, and J. P. Roll. Op. cit.

[43] Valera, F. Op. cit.

[44] Sakurai, Y, 1996. Op. cit.

[45] Moore, Keith, and T. Persaud. *The Developing Human,* 6th ed. (Philadelphia: W. B. Saunders, 1996), 87, 427.

[46] Comeaux, Zachary. Op. cit.

[47] Becker, Robert. *The Body Electric: Electromagnetism and the Foundation of Life* (New York: William Morrow, 1985), 72.

Chapter 9

FOR—Basic Concepts

A Dynamic Method of Neuromuscular and Ligamentous/Articular Assessment and Treatment

Facilitated Oscillatory Release (FOR) is a method for applying oscillatory force in a treatment sequence intended to normalize muscle tone and articular balance in traumatized or strained tissue. FOR has been expressed initially in an osteopathic context but not as a proprietary or free-standing modality. It has been mostly integrated into the focal treatment style popular with American osteopaths, as an adjunct to high-velocity low-amplitude (HVLA), muscle energy (MET), or connective tissue release techniques. My prejudice is that the common ground in most methods of bodywork is the relationship of the practitioner to the patient's connective tissue system. In this spirit, the concepts can complement many types of bodywork. As reviewed in the scientific literature in the preceding chapter, I suggest that rhythmic peripheral afferent input can enable the resetting of normal postural muscle tone. The associated neurophysiological theory and research may help further validate osteopathic diagnosis and treatment, and the nature of what has been termed somatic dysfunction, on a fundamental level.

As a clinician and teacher, I have experienced that the approach described here works and is appreciated by students. However, having a limited ability to test the hypothesis of effectiveness through instrumentation, I rely heavily on the synopsis of supportive research previously presented. Correlation with this material will be made as appropriate. Clearly there is work to be done and further literature to be examined to refine, emend, or dismiss the current hypothesis.

Although not essential for basic application, the suggested theory of effectiveness involves a decreasing of problematic muscle tone through entrainment of the body's own rhythmically firing neuroproprioceptive system. Coordinative processing of afferent input, which is preliminary to an active response, has been modeled as a coding process. As noted before, neuronal population coding has challenged or replaced modular and line labeled coordination in much of the neurophysiological literature.[1,2,3] It is a challenge then for the clinician to incorporate the implications of this further research into practice to increase the benefit to the patient.

Developmental Background

Any method of approach in bodywork optimally should integrate art, science, and clinical experience. Each element expands our capacity for enlightened intervention in patient care. FOR blends these modes in using rhythmic repetitive motion of body parts to help in diagnosis and in normalization of function. Most other osteopathic methods use a minimal if any amount of rhythm in motion testing despite the importance of rhythmic motion in daily function (walking, cycling, running). Exceptions have been noted in Chapter 3. Methods of bodywork that use rhythmic motion, other than FOR, do not include the precision of osteopathic diagnosis. Specific localization to a target tissue enhances and optimizes the intended effect by precisely directing force as well as the intention to heal.

As implied in the trend of thought developed in Chapter 8, rate, location, and temporal associations of signals have been cited as key features of the functional activity of the neural system. Several researchers have seen patterns of cyclic depolarization-repolarization activity as the body's means of sensing, interpreting, and responding to external stimuli.[4,5] In a separate area of work, symptoms such as pain are often seen as due to the diffusion and retention of the energy of strain or traumatic contact.[6,7,8] As noted in Chapter 5, Giselher Schalow has used repetitive afferent impulses of the correct resonant frequency therapeutically to relieve muscle tension and restore comfort and function.[9] Fulford used percussive vibration in a compatible fashion. Consistent with this research, FOR is suggested to be a means of manually applying therapeutic rhythmic force in a convenient way to restore motion and reduce pain.[10]

I was trained as an American osteopathic physician and have maintained an interest in traditional and classical osteopathic philosophy and methods. A variety of treatment models (articular, muscle energy, HVLA, counterstrain, myofascial release) have been derived from the experience of astute clinicians. Attempts at physiological modeling have been progressive since the beginning of osteopathy; however, explanations have lagged well behind clinical practice and research. Most models depend on properties of articular mechanics[11,12] and classical neuromuscular control.[13,14] Initially during student days, through the instigation of Anthony Chila, DO, I was teased to incorporate techniques and observations outside of, or inconsistent with, the classical osteopathic paradigm. FOR has been formalized from my practice style as a result of my quest to reconcile these elements. This chapter will present background thought and principles. Examples of application drills as well as integration into actual practice will be found in Chapters 10, 11, and 12.

As mentioned above, I was also exposed to the person, thought, and practice of Robert Fulford, DO, who expounded a unique expression of cranial osteopathy influenced by Randolph Stone, DO,[15] and others. Fulford redefined the patient according to vibrational electromagnetic field theory to complement his biomechanical training. Encouraged by readings in neurophysiological research, and personal exploration, Fulford evolved a protocol using oscillatory force and described his methods in terms of an energetic model. Part of treatment for Fulford was the use of a mechanical vibratory force (percussion vibrator) to release the shock of trauma remaining in damaged or painful tissue.[16] As a result of this teaching exposure, I integrated these procedures into the pattern of osteopathic manipulative treatment, and searched further for an understanding of tissue characteristics compatible with field theory, yet also compatible with more widely accepted neurophysiology and biomechanics. Additionally, I sought a manual means for the dynamic application of vibratory force in a clinically efficient way, independent of the percussion vibrator. Besides the convenience, this would help bridge the ideological chasm between energetic and conventional manipulation.

In actual practice, FOR is seen to complement other methods of diagnosis and treatment and is used in combined treatments. The procedures described in this text are intended to be exercises to help the reader become sensitized to the means and issues in applying rhythmic force to a body with therapeutic intent. Individual implementation in practice can vary.

Universality of Rhythmic Motion, Macroscopic and Microscopic

Joggers and cyclists experience the natural feel and function of rhythm. Babies appreciate being rocked when unhappy; many of us dance for joy. None of this is incidental. Rhythmic motion is everywhere in human experience. Just as biologists recognize diurnal and other rhythms, much of function, even on a microscopic scale, is rhythmic. On the level of physiological function, respiration and cardiac function are commonly recognized to be rhythmic. But voluntary and involuntary movements are commonly seen as the result of discrete linear and sequential processes. However, on a microscopic level, as we have seen in the physiological review above, movement and maintenance of postural tone reflect recurrent cyclic depolarization and repolarization of the muscle activation pathway that extend the event from one of milliseconds to the time scale of purposeful gross motion.[17] Muscle function is, then, also biochemically rhythmic following this cycle of depolarization-repolarization.

As noted above, both the counterstrain and muscle energy models of manipulation make mention of the hypothesis of Korr and the inappropriate balance of gamma and alpha motor neuron activity present in dysfunction.[18] This began to expand osteopathic thought beyond the concept of spinal facilitation, which emphasized the level of neural connectivity to one of altered peripheral proprioceptive function. The emphasis in the FOR model is also on the functional coordination or traffic pattern on these pathways. It relies heavily on the concepts of neural coding and depolarization by resonant cell assemblies, described in Chapter 8.

The information on the effectiveness and theoretical basis for tonic vibratory reflex is of special relevance in building up the idea of entrainment of proprioceptive coordination. This special relevance derives in part from the coincidence in application of resonance in Fulford's percussion vibrator model.

The bringing together of the research in tonic vibratory reflex, resonant cell assemblies, and temporospatial neural coding seemed to me to contribute to the explanation of the clinical effects of percussive vibratory and FOR application of external oscillatory force. This literature also suggests a new direction to go in our appreciation of the neuromuscular component of hypertonic muscle, as well as joint position and tenderness, in models of somatic dysfunction generally.

Rationale for Extending the Use of Manual Oscillatory Effect on Tissues

Many somatic complaints resulting from musculoskeletal trauma or strain involve asymmetric muscle tone associated with restriction of motion and positional asymmetries of bony parts. If voluntary and proprioceptive muscle function involve rhythmic neural coordination in health, as is suggested by numerous investigators, it would seem logical to pursue an understanding of the associated dysrhythmias in musculoskeletal pain syndromes. It seems plausible to hypothesize the hypertonic muscle tissue so frequently associated with pain and dysfunction as representing a dysfunctionally altered baseline rhythmic state of depolarization, a dysrhythmia. If not a sustained dysrhythmia, it may well have begun with an incomplete or functionally inappropriate rhythmic coordinative initiating event. In either case, based on the tonic vibratory reflex and percussion vibration data, the hypertonia may be altered by the application of a functionally appropriate rhythmic force. This may milk edema fluid from the area, may directly stretch tissue, may gently rearrange joint surfaces, or, more to the point, may induce, through entrainment, a functionally appropriate level of oscillatory neural coordination. In an articular or myofascial manipulation context, it may be an occasion to add energy to that had been lost through trauma in order to reverse the deformation of connective tissue through hysteresis.

All these are included in the intention of FOR, when applied in the context of a general protocol of manipulation. It is my perception that many models of treatment complement one another in practice, and that effective treatment is most often eclectic or a combination therapy, due to the multivariate cause in many physiological problems. FOR is to be thought of in this manner.

More particularly, FOR represents a dynamic and expedient method of connective tissue normalization. Consequently, just as connective tissue stretch is part of preparation and localization in many treatment approaches, including articular, high-velocity low-amplitude, and muscle energy treatments, FOR is most practically combined with these methods during the localization phase to increase the effectiveness of all techniques. However, as one recognizes the effect of FOR, and some of the peculiar advantages it possesses, one can develop maneuvers in which the role of oscillatory function begins to predominate as the effective force.

Propagation of a Wave

To effectively apply oscillatory force in tissue, it helps to be familiar with or recall certain basic concepts of wave propagation in any physical medium.

Force applied to a medium is dispersed in a pattern concentric from the source. Waves propagate until they meet resistance. Resistance due to friction over a distance, or other obstacles in the medium, may dampen or diminish the amplitude of the wave.

The displacements in the medium by two or more waves have an effect on one another.

Two waves in a medium may be in phase (coinciding their peaks, valleys, and crossover nodes) or out of phase. Waves generated by rhythmic force create a series of waves (wave trains). Individual or wave trains that coincide with each other with displacements in the same direction will reinforce each other and add their amplitudes of displacement of the medium (constructive interference). Waves or wave trains that coincide with each other but having displacements in the opposite direction will compete and decrease the amplitude of the composite displacement of the medium (destructive interference). Any degree of difference in phase leads to partial interference with proportionate effects.

On reaching a medium of different density, the force of a wave incident on the new surface is either transmitted or reflected, depending on the relative densities of the two media and the angle of incidence. If transmitted, the energy of the wave enters the new medium. If reflected, the reflected wave, if in phase with the incident wave, will reinforce it and if the initiating force is continued, will maintain what is called a standing wave. As children, many of us enjoyed creating waves in a bathtub, dishpan, or other body of water until we got a higher and higher splash, an example of developing a standing wave.

Entrainment is the phenomenon in which one wave pattern, either because of strength or persistence, causes another wave to adopt the frequency and phase of the initial wave. A classic example is the way in which sound waves from ticking clocks in a clock shop, caused by swinging pendulums, will drift toward synchrony under the influence of the most powerful clock.

Application of Wave Propagation in Body Tissues

So what does this have to do with working with body tissue? How can we effectively apply all this theory? The linear elements of fascia and muscle hold certain tension as a result of forces acting upon them. In the bodywork context we can create conditions that may adjust or tune the tension in these tissues. Strain and dysfunction represent an imbalance in tensions. Treatment involves returning the tissue, region, or system to balance. One can tune a guitar as an artist, or as an engineer. Most instruments are tuned by the musician—by ear, not by a scientist with instrumentation, despite our ability to describe music in scientific acoustical terms. As bodyworkers we focus on selective areas of the body, including particular "target issues," and can use this tuning analogy as we work by feel, judgment, analysis, and intuition. The ideas can be integrated with many existing methods, or can follow a prescribed protocol. I realize that the composite of tissues of the body is remarkably complex. But most methods of bodywork attempt to isolate particular tissues, including linear arrangements, in order to have a desired effect.

Much of the work that follows is done in the spirit of such an artist who would work by feel with the body as an instrument, as responsive to oscillatory force. Once one understands these rhythmic characteristics of tissue, one can work with what one feels and judges to be the appropriate or inappropriate application of oscillatory force, and make adjustment as one sees fit. Again, the instrument tuning analogy seems most appropriate.

Many of the tissue elements of the body, especially in the musculoskeletal system, have linearly arranged fibers. Striated muscle and their supportive fascias, responsible for voluntary and postural stabilization, have such directional lines, parallel to the direction of contraction. As such, they are capable of transmitting vibratory force, and resonating in response to this force as a plucked guitar string. Additionally, force applied along the lengths of the fibers to their attachment points can transmit force to the more solid elements of the skeletal system. Ease of dispersion of force through the tissue, location of dampening especially comparing paired or serial elements such as spinal vertebrae, or paired extremities, can localize dysfunction. With experience, the characteristics of reflection or transmission of force at origins and insertions can all be used diagnostically to identify dysfunction.

Consider the spinal vertebral musculature. If the short musculature such as the multifidi, interspinatus, and transversarii are implicated in a pattern of segmental[19] dysfunction, cyclic rotatory motion will repetitively stretch and potentially activate muscle spindles and nociceptive afferents involved with these muscles. The role of this activation will be described in more detail in Chapter 12. Additionally, the result of strain or trauma may, through compression and distortion of connective tissue, result in the absorption then dissipation of the energy of an applied force (hysteresis), leaving tissue distortion.[20] An example may be an inversion sprain to an ankle. Theoretically, the gentle application of oscillatory force may partially reverse the deformation retained in tissue and accelerate restoration of integrity of structure, and therefore of function. It would be appropriate to view this as restoring endogenous energy lost through hysteresis, or dissipating the shock of trauma.[21] Both solid elements and fluid components create the rigidity and turgor to transmit this energy through tissue.[22]

Sustained oscillatory force, in the form of a standing wave, can be used to diagnose, and the force can then be modified to mobilize local dampening, articular restriction, or inappropriate hypertonia in muscle. The strategy for intervention may vary. For significant restriction, especially involving articular restriction to motion, an abrupt variation of the phase of oscillatory force of the standing wave, creating a destructive interference pattern, may be necessary to distort the connective tissue matrix to its native, pre-injury state. Another strategy is to alter the tone in muscle fibers under unnecessary adaptive tension by a gentle but firm application of oscillatory force, to induce a new harmonic resonant pattern (entrainment). This often leads to a release of tension and a restoration of tissue relaxation. The same application of force may be imparted to tissue to add energy at the origin or insertion, to affect the state of ligaments, articular capsules, or articular surfaces. The strategy is much like jiggling the tumblers in a lock in which the key will not turn, as an alternative to twisting with more force to overcome resistance.

The application of these strategies will be developed below as exercises in beginning to play with, and tame, the use of oscillatory force for integration into clinical practice.

References

[1] Sakurai, Y. "How do cell assemblies encode information in the brain?" *Neurosci Biobehav Rev*, 23(6), 1999, 785–796.

[2] Sanger, T. D. "Neural population codes," *Curr Opin Neurobiol*, 13(2), 2003, 238–249.

[3] Doetsch, G. S. "Patterns in the brain: Neuronal population coding in the somatosensory system," *Physiol Behav*, 69(1–2), 2000, 187–201.

[4] Farmer, S. "Rhythmicity, synchronization and binding in human and primate motor systems," *J Physiol*, 509(1), 1998, 3–14.

[5] Zedka, M. "Phasic activity in the human erector spinae during repetitive hand motions," *J Physiol*, 504(3), 1997, 727–734.

[6] Upledger, John. *Somatoemotional Release and Beyond* (Berkeley, Calif.: North Atlantic Books, 2002).

[7] Comeaux, Zachary. *Robert Fulford, DO, and the Philosopher Physician* (Seattle: Eastland Press, 2002).

[8] Becker, Robert. *The Body Electric: Electromagnetism and the Foundation of Life* (New York: William Morrow, 1985).

[9] Schalow, Giselher. "Spinal oscillators in man under normal and pathological conditions," *Electromyog Clin Neurophysio*, (33), 1993, 409–426.

[10] Comeaux, Zachary. "Facilitated Oscillatory Release: A method of dynamic assessment and treatment of somatic dysfunction," *American Academy of Osteopathy Journal*, 13(3), 2003, 30–35.

[11] Fryette, Harrison. *Principles of Osteopathic Technique* (Kirksville, Mo.: Journal Printing Company, 1994).

[12] Hall, T. E., and John Wernham. *The Contribution of J M Littlejohn to Osteopathy* (Maidstone, England: Maidstone Osteopathic Clinic, 1974).

[13] Jones, Lawrence. *Jones Strain CounterStrain*, 2nd ed. (Boise: Jones Strain-CounterStrain Inc, 1995).

[14] Mitchell, Fred. *The Muscle Energy Manual*, vol. 1. (East Lansing, Mich.: MET Press, 1995).

[15] Stone, Randolph. *Polarity Therapy* (Sebastopol, Calif.: CRCS Publications, 1987).

[16] Comeaux, Zachary, 2002. Op. cit.

[17] McComas, Alan. *Skeletal Muscle: Form and Function* (Champaign, Ill.: Human Kinetics, 1996).

[18] Korr, Irwin. "Proprioceptors and somatic dysfunction," *Journal of the American Osteopathic Association*, (74), 1975, 638–650.

[19] Mitchell, Fred. Op. cit.

[20] Lederman, Eyal. *Fundamental of Manual Therapy: Physiology, Neurology and Psychology* (New York: Churchill Livingston, 1997).

[21] Becker, Robert. Op. cit.

[22] Lederman, Eyal. Op. cit.

Chapter 10

Application of FOR Principles

Application Exercises—Spine

The reader should remember the context of this sharing, and realize that the exercises described here do not represent complete diagnostic or treatment recommendations. In this chapter, the exercises are drill activities to begin giving one a feel for the use of rhythmic force in treatment. Chapters 11 and 12 give examples of clinical application. However, even here they need to be applied and integrated into the context of the practitioner's training, license, and practice setting. This is most directly done in the context of osteopathic practice, as will be described at the beginning of Chapter 11, but the principles may be adopted in many settings.

Many of the exercises and treatments are presented in the context of diagnosing and treating in relation to a restrictive barrier. The concept initially describes the anatomical limits of motion of tissue or a joint, beyond which damage occurs if distention is forced. Within this range of anatomical motion, there is a physiological range of motion. If there is a limitation within this physiological range of normal function, we term it a restrictive barrier. Reestablishing the full range of physiological function is the goal of treatment.

Rhythmic activities are a natural way our bodies seek to conserve or restore normal function.

One goal of good bodywork is to remember that we are trying to restore normal function. The value of natural activities, such as walking or jogging, is recognized in this regard.

The stretch, cyclic afferent input, and articulatory movements associated with natural gait are a useful way of mobilizing restricted segments of the central axis. The FOR approach to the spine and sacrum attempts to replicate aspects of the gait cycle involving the axial skeleton and its supportive tissue. Beginning with the patient in a prone position, the practitioner uses oscillation by initiating a gentle, continuous rocking of the pelvis with the caudal-most hand, alternately from side to side using one hand. The heel or fingertips of the other hand, reaching across the spine, are placed over a transverse process of the vertebrae. This hand is then set into motion rhythmically in phase with the motion of the pelvis, but going in the opposite direction, thus creating torsion of the torso. In other words, as the hand on the pelvis moves away from the practitioner, that adjacent to the spine moves toward; at the end of that excursion, the directions are reversed in each hand.

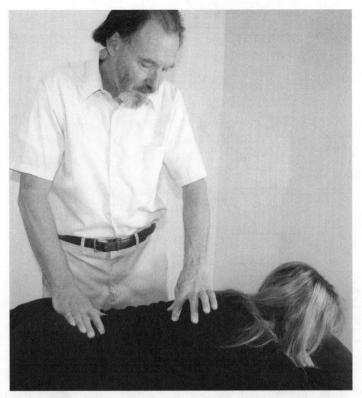

Figure 10-1. Reciprocal rotational motion is developed in
a body part of some mass to create a standing wave effect,
which is transmitted regionally. Here, the pelvis is rotated to
transmit force through the trunk.

The uppermost hand adjacent to the spine will now be given
a second role, that of simultaneously assessing the quality of
response in the tissues to the induced motion. Once a person can
begin to read the tissue in this manner, he or she can then move
the sensing upper hand up and down the spine to compare the
response at various specific spinal segments. With practice, one
develops a sense of a normal rhythmic compliance. Comparison
to segments above and below can isolate segments that are less
than optimally compliant. Clinical correlation will help decide

the involvement of such a segment with symptoms. This protocol involves passive motion testing and primarily the rotational phase of motion, but assesses also the general tone in the local region. Dysfunction is perceived as a dysrhythmic response to the induced motion.

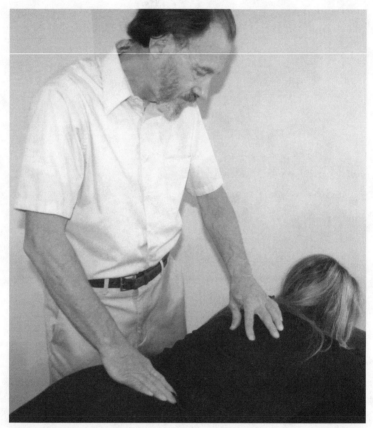

Figure 10-2. Moving fingers along the spine assesses the comparative response of each segment to oscillation.

If the practitioner discovers localized dysfunction in this manner, he or she can restore or facilitate optimal resonance, rhythmic compliance, and freedom of motion by one of three strategies of application of rhythmic force.

One strategy is to induce a stretch or articulation mobilization with a rapid exaggeration of the rotation of the segment in phase with the anticipated oscillation. This would represent a situation of constructive interference with the induced standing wave of force previously initiated in the tissues. A second, more forceful strategy is to add the exaggerated rotation out of phase with the developed rhythm. This applies a destructive interference pattern to the established wave in the tissue by introducing more energy. A third intervention strategy is to gently persist with the established wave pattern to soften tissue by inducing any resistance in the tissue to accept the energy of the new wave pattern. This allows the rhythmic afferent input to entrain a more homeostatic endogenous rhythm of the neurons responsible for coordinating postural tone. In this application the intent would be to induce a relaxation pattern of baseline neuromuscular coordination and to entrain a more harmonic pattern.

Using the musical instrument analogy, the work is much like playing a stringed instrument and sliding on the neck to create notes, as in a dobro, slide guitar, or pedal steel guitar.

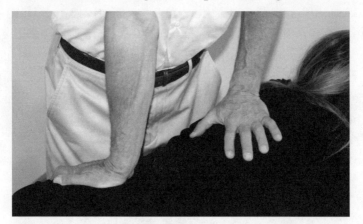

Figure 10-3. Heel of hand or thumb is ready to transmit corrective force during oscillation, either in phase or out of phase with the standing wave, and depending on intent.

If a practitioner is applying these strategies to the spine, it is wise to begin with the patient in as gravity-neutral a posture as possible, yet with access to the spine. The prone position meets these conditions and is recommended. In this manner, a pattern of passive activity and afferent stimulation is reproduced that is equivalent to that during active walking, with its alternating pelvic rotation and counter torsion through the trunk. Once assimilated, it is possible to transfer most of these strategies to the seated position. This is done very effectively in the GOT (general osteopathic treatment) taught and practiced by John Wernham as a classical technique. Treatment in the lateral recumbent position is also possible.

As described thus far, in the prone position the thoracic and lumbar spine are treated by rotating the pelvis to develop a standing wave, and adding counter torsion of the trunk, with localization as necessary. To diagnose and treat in the pelvis and more particularly the sacrum, a reciprocal role of the two hands is used by rotating the trunk to generate momentum and letting the sacral hand "listen" to the quality and quantity of resonant tissue compliance and to then make corrective suggestion (see Figure 10-4). I find this strategy most useful after diagnosing the pelvic area by other means, usually using the parameters of the muscle energy model. Then, in the prone position, the oscillatory force may be applied to the most posterior dysfunctional surface of the sacrum.

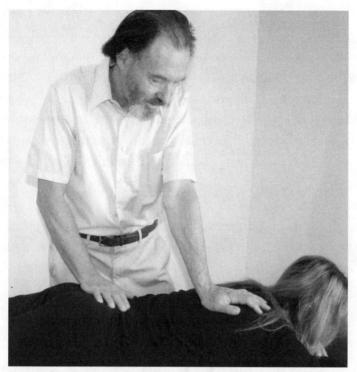

Figure 10-4. In sacral or pelvic treatment, the roles of the oscillating and monitoring hand are reversed. The trunk is oscillated to direct motion to the pelvic region.

In osteopathic or muscle energy treatment context, an example would be in treatment of a left unilateral flexion of the sacrum by applying contact to the inferior lateral angle on the left. This would be the most posterior aspect of the sacrum.[1] Attention would be paid to staying clear of the coccyx. Once the oscillatory pattern of motion is established through the trunk, a firm counter pressure in phase, or at 180 degrees out of phase, to the cycle of the thoracic rotation could be applied for reasons mentioned in the description of thoracolumbar spine treatment. Similarly, if the diagnosis were a left on left sacral torsion, with the problem being an anterior right sacral base, the contact hand would be placed over the left inferior lateral angle, the most posterior prominence. To treat an extended sacrum, such as a left on right torsion, a slightly more elaborate strategy is necessary. Pressure is placed over the posterior left sacral base with firm thumb pressure. But to create the potential for motion, the practitioner gaps the sacro-iliac joint by using the patient's leg on a bent knee for leverage. The operator internally rotates the thigh to open the SI joint. The same leverage is used to initially oscillate the pelvis using one's upper torso. Should this force not be adequate, passive anterior rotation of the innominate is added to coax the adjacent sacral base to move anteriorly. Application of an active isometric contraction of the patient in hip flexion can complete the effort. For further clarification of integration with muscle energy technique, see Figures 11-1 and 11-2.

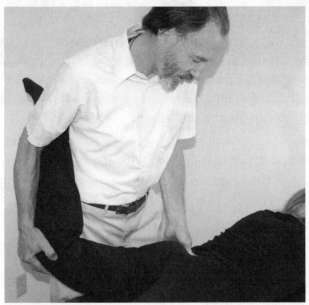

Figure 10-5. Applying pressure to the most posterior aspect of the sacrum, the practitioner uses the lower extremity for leverage and introduces oscillation with the rhythmic sway of his or her own body mass.

Application Exercises—Extremities

As will be discussed below, oscillatory force may be used with specific intent in a number of diagnostic and treatment contexts. The lower extremities and pelvis represent a complex region. Here the use of oscillation will be described in a more general way in order to allow the reader to get a feel for using this type of force.

By suspending the lower extremity in the supine patient (with practitioner at the foot of the table), then cupping the heel and comparing the response to subtle rocking motion from side to side, a practitioner may form an impression of the degree and location of any general regional restriction. Depending on one's palpatory sensitivity, one can surmise fascial or articular restriction of motion within the leg, thigh, or pelvis and select a tissue to be targeted for treatment. The practitioner may add further refinements in the following ways. Grasping the ankle by surrounding the limb with the hands, the practitioner first applies traction and torsion to the extremity to localize the effect of the motion to be introduced to further discriminate the level needing attention. Traction is best applied using one's body weight, leaning backwards, to exert firm but gentle force along the long axis of the leg. Additional therapeutic force is then applied by creating oscillation of the extremity by alternately raising and lowering one's arms using shoulder strength, in a pumping motion, at 60–100 cycles per minute. Speed is determined by the resonant response of the tissues of the extremity and will vary with the proportions, age, and physical characteristics of the patient. One does what feels right, smooth, and responsive. Oscillatory motion can alternatively be directed in the patient's coronal plane.

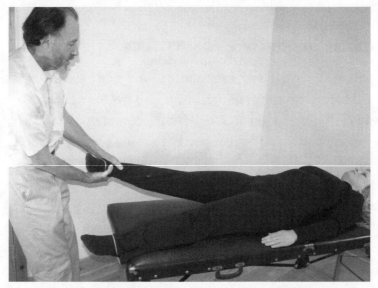

Figure 10-6. Connective tissue is first put under tension to transmit corrective force. Spiral torsions can be induced to carry the localization farther from the point of contact.

This continues until there is a release, or a judgment that further release is not likely to occur. Ten seconds is usually more than enough time to develop the effect desired. This approach differs from Harmonic Release technique in which cephalad/caudad oscillation is commonly used in the latter with a different conceptualization of localization.

In the upper extremity, FOR is best applied in the context of, or extension of, connective tissue or myofascial release. Diagnostic oscillation can be applied regionally to the "long lever" of the upper extremity with the patient in a supine position, by wrapping one hand around the patient's wrist, the other just distal to the area under study. Here we are describing traction to the supine patient, with the arm abducted. Again, using his or her body weight, the practitioner may apply gentle traction with additional torsion as logical, while grasping the wrist to pre-stretch tissues. Vibration is created by rhythmically raising and lowering one's arms, thereby transferring an oscillatory wave through the extremity. See Figure 10-7 to clarify the position. Most often, inclusion of the shoulder girdle in diagnosis and treatment is essential. Sensitivity to myofascial tension in this area can be maximized by spiraling the fascia of the arm in internal rotation. In this manner, the arm and forearm become more rigid, and the most responsive parts are the glenohumeral joint, the acromioclavicular and sternoclavicular joints, and the thoracoscapular attachment, and their supportive soft tissue. We can add abduction and flexion of the limb at the glenohumeral joint, according to need. Stereognostic palpation can help localize the area of greatest resistance to resonance, or dampening of the standing wave we create to test, and therapeutic oscillation can be directed to the tissues responsible for this restriction.

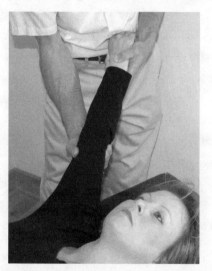

Figure 10-7. Myofascial traction can be used strategically to localize the effect of oscillatory force. Rhythmic motion is induced at a rate dependent on the distance between attachments and resonant characteristics of the tissue under treatment.

The reader may visualize what is intended by stereognostic palpation with the following example. If blindfolded, and holding out a pencil by grasping it at each end, consider the palpatory experience of a colleague offering a fulcrum for rotation, a rigid finger, somewhere along the length of the pencil. From the different data gathered from each hand, the reader could estimate or mentally visualize, without actually seeing, the location of the fulcrum. With various trials, the palpatory sense would become more refined. So it is with clinical palpation. In many situations, direct visualization of a restriction is not possible or inconclusive. Clinical judgment is enhanced by the information gained from various passive motion tests. Clinical success and failure direct the refinement of the palpatory assessment process.

Gentle oscillatory force coupled with connective tissue tension can promote further specificity in localizing restriction of motion, leading to more focused treatment strategies. Using the strategy of directing oscillatory force from an operating hand generating the movement to a hand directed toward the restriction, one can place the hands at any location of restriction in the arm. The practitioner's operating forearm can then be rapidly internally and externally rotated in a tremulous fashion, to generate the oscillatory force required. In this way one can work with the fascias, focusing on the carpal retinaculum, the interosseous membrane, the biceps and triceps musculature, the pectoralis, levator scapulae, or rotator cuff muscles, separately or together.

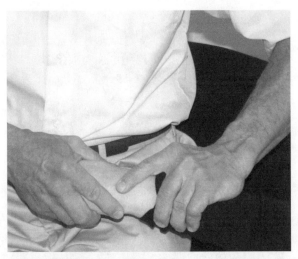

Figure 10-8. Shorter distance between the practitioner's hands allows for more precision in correction. Here, attention is paid to the wrist.

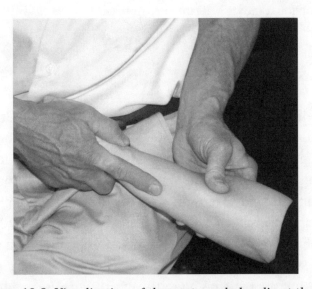

Figure 10-9. Visualization of the anatomy helps direct the force to the intended tissue—here, the interosseus membrane between radius and ulna.

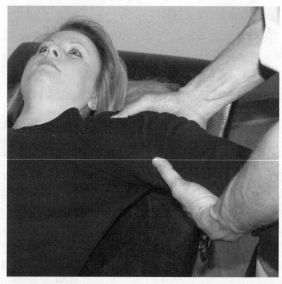

Figure 10-10. The complex anatomy of the shoulder in the glenohumeral joint can be treated by sequentially changing the amount and vector of tension to assess then treat individual muscles, ligaments, and fascias.

Other Applications

Focal neuro-inhibition has been used as a treatment for increased myotonia for more than a hundred years.[2] In the FOR context, using the index finger to locally direct the application of force and the same hand and forearm to generate a wave, oscillation can be directed to such focal tension points as the atlanto-occipital area, the iliotibial band, or a costochondral area. See Figure 10-11. As in the application of the forearm just described, rather than generating the standing wave by the practitioner's movement of some mass within the patient's body, the practitioner uses some part of his or her own body. In instances such as this focal application, there is no body part of the patient to act as the lever in creating and maintaining momentum for the standing wave. So, in this case the momentum is initiated in the practitioner, with a node of the wave corresponding to the point of contact. From this contact point the force is disseminated to the intended tissues. Further permutations in applying the principles of FOR will be addressed under the integration of techniques in Chapter 12.

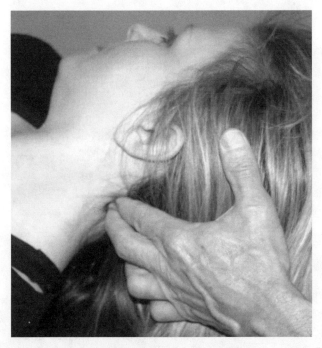

Figure 10-11. Precise direction of force can be transmitted through the fingertip in contact with the tissue to be treated.

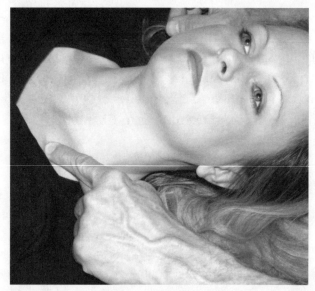

Figure 10-12. In fingertip localization, the standing wave is created using the practitioner's forearm as the oscillating mass, the fingertip at the node of the wave, the force being transmitted to the adjacent tissues of the patient.

References

[1] Mitchell, Fred. *The Muscle Energy Manual,* vol. 1 (East Lansing, Mich.: MET Press, 1995).

[2] Olmstead, J. *Charles Edouard Brown-Seguard: Nineteenth Century Neurologist and Endocrinologist* (Baltimore: Johns Hopkins University Press, 1946).

Chapter 11

FOR Integration in Clinical Practice

Adaptation to Practice Context

As has been noted, the exercises described here are not necessarily actual practice protocols as much as examples of application of certain principles involving corrective, facilitative force. However, they may be adapted as protocols as the situation warrants. More typically, oscillatory force is used to nuance a previously described technique, or to challenge anatomically identified, problematic tissue. Each case is an individual physiological problem to be solved with the principles presented here, plus the practitioner's insight, experience, and ingenuity. What is the target tissue, how has it arrived in its current state, and what does it need to resume normal function?

Osteopathy, as bodywork in general, represents a family of approaches. In the words of A. T. Still, there is no one way to treat, to return the unnatural to the natural. As a result, each practitioner will select different principles and apply them in a unique manner. As mentioned before, I was trained as an American osteopathic physician, in which context certain models have been formalized and several protocols in each model standardized. However, like many other practitioners, I choose to practice in an eclectic style of combined technique with any one patient and session. Several descriptive scenarios, derived from my practice and building on biomechanical approaches, are included here to inspire the reader's creativity and encourage exploration.

Adaptation to Patient Position and Clinical Task

The number of applications of FOR are limited only by one's imagination and clinical experience. They may be integrated into a wide variety of clinical situations. However, one thing we have not mentioned so far is the practitioner's posture and demeanor. In applying these techniques, the practitioner must be relaxed, with a stable base, grounded and balanced but not rigid. To create the oscillating force, one must have an effective contact, but equally important is the attitude. The rhythm should flow naturally, as in dance, intentional but not forced. The natural resonance of the tissue under treatment should help a practitioner "get a feel for the music."

In the setup for a traditional lateral recumbent lumbar thrust technique, while the patient's torso is placed supine and stabilized with the practitioner's most cephalad arm or hand, the lower extremity and pelvis are rotated toward the practitioner and allowed to go beyond the table edge, to generate torque in the lower lumbar spine. Figure 11-1 clarifies the setup. The practitioner's free hand or forearm is used to accentuate this rotation and to localize to the articulation intended for treatment. Once the range of initial passive motion is reached, one can use steadily applied connective tissue stretch to optimize effective localization of force to the segments to which treatment is intended. Should one want to improve effectiveness by introducing an isometric contraction against resistance, further release may be attained and the restrictive barrier may be more closely approximated. Thus far one has used connective tissue stretch plus muscle energy. In this context of stacking methods to optimize advantage, the practitioner may add gentle oscillation by rocking the torso, while emphasizing the stretch through the lower, thrusting arm, applied to the thigh or ileum, to further improve release prior to or after the thrust. Often, the thrust will be superfluous.

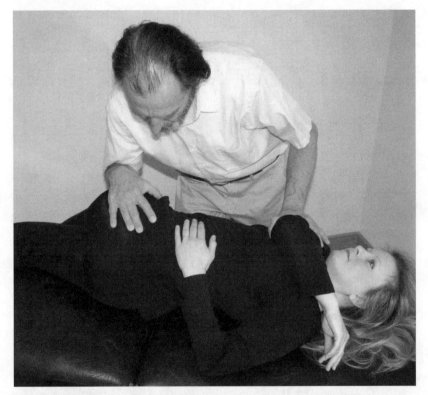

Figure 11-1. FOR can be integrated into any treatment position in which a barrier to motion is conceptualized. Here, we position for muscle energy lumbar treatment.

Similarly, if one intends to apply a muscle energy (MET) treatment to an anteriorly rotated innominate, by flexing the ipsilateral hip, anticipating isometric contraction of the hip extensor to rotate the pelvis, the same sequence of connective tissue stretch and isometric contraction may be enhanced by integrating oscillatory rocking of the loaded pelvis, in the same plane as the other forces, both before and after the applied isometric contraction.

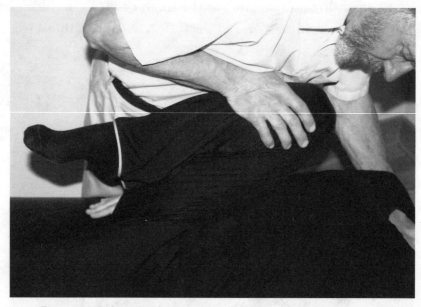

Figure 11-2. In muscle energy technique, the barrier is approached. Rhythmic oscillation, in addition to relaxed exhalation, helps advance the restricted barrier more gently, quickly, and completely.

If the problem in the pelvic region is a sacral one, with bilateral restriction in flexion or extension (unilateral restriction was addressed above in the text at Figure 10-4), the sacrum may be cupped with the patient prone and simultaneously rocked rhythmically from side to side, coupled with the desired articular flexion or extension, as appropriate.

The rudimentary prone spinal exercise described at the beginning of Chapter 10 may be executed as a seated treatment since the buttocks, being fixed to the treatment table, provide resistance to rhythmic rotation or sidebending of the trunk. This is similar to what is done in the GOT of Wernham.

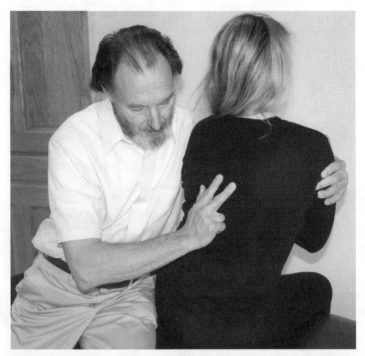

Figure 11-3. This setup replicates the seated assessment style of John Wernham in application of general osteopathic technique, a method compatible with FOR.

It may be added, however, that from this position one can easily proceed to Functional Methods technique, counterstrain, or muscle energy, without repositioning the patient. FOR may be sufficient by itself, or may precondition the patient to be receptive to the subsequent method of treatment.

Adaptation to Clinical Goals

Chronic overuse syndromes of the upper extremity are notoriously difficult to resolve by any means. Onset is insidious and may result in various degrees of thoracic outlet syndrome, brachial neuritis, and carpal tunnel syndrome. The advantage of manipulative approaches over conservative or surgical approaches is modest but significant. Any approach relies on specificity of intervention. The difficulty in treating these conditions is very often due to the multivariate causes and the complexity of the region, so that the restriction is not limited to one specific location. Hence the classical usage of such phrases as double or triple crush syndrome in neuro-orthopedic literature.

A connective tissue approach begins by surveying the whole shoulder and thoracic region to gather tactile feedback regarding the state of the tissues. Tension is palpable. Often we introduce the force required to resolve the results of tissue strain as a gentle stretch. Sometimes a more forceful stretch is required, often over repetitive applications in successive sessions. Adding oscillation has several advantages. First, the activating, remediating force is introduced repetitively in the single session, with the potential to accelerate change. Additionally, the feedback one gets from this successive introduction of force can refine the localization of the point of maximal restriction; it also allows one to advance toward a primary cause as secondary restrictions fade under the healing oscillatory stretch. The process is very much like unraveling a complex knot in a rope. As first the tight knots seem dauntingly complex and impossible to untie. But by gentle and clever persistence, complex knots and tangles can be undone. So with the results of trauma and strain, tissues in unnatural configurations can be coaxed to resume their resting state through gentle rhythmic force.

The speed and cadence of FOR have another advantage to the practitioner, especially in early stages of learning. In much myofascial work or connective tissue work, it takes an act of faith to believe that one is working with the body and working some good, especially in the slow unwinding or indirect methods. The dialogue with the body is subtle, and with a slow cadence, the feedback that one is achieving a result is sometimes slow to come. With this delay it is often difficult to associate one's efforts with the results, whatever they may be. In FOR, the rhythm itself is gentle and easily accepted by the body. The rate and force of application can progress more rapidly, more directly, without becoming intrusive to the patient. As a result, feedback is quick. There is a more proximate association of one's effort and the results. It is as if the session is a biofeedback protocol in which one is successively guided by the evolving state of the tissues.

This reminds me of the hard work of hand-sanding old furniture to refinish it. The rhythmic effort of applying the sandpaper takes effort and a certain faith in the results. As the wood grain emerges from the old finish, one can recognize the qualities and see the potential in the piece being refinished. It guides the refinisher to modify but persist in efforts. There is immediate feedback. So it is with the dynamic application of connective tissue release in FOR.

Recently I had a case of a woman who had aching and numbness in one arm with a developing problem in the other. The woman worked as a cashier in a grocery, pushing items past her cash register all day. She was a large woman, with a full chest and broad shoulders with very developed upper-extremity musculature. She was overweight, with central obesity suggesting some degree of adrenal dysregulation. Her mother had surgery for carpal tunnel syndrome. Clearly her problems were multifactorial and the case represented a challenge.

The case is relevant here because, after clearing her of cervical foraminal impingement, there were limited results to conventional manipulation over several sessions, using primarily linear and spiral stretch to the potential levels of impingement in the extremities: the pectoralis, the supraspinatus, the scalene muscle, first rib, triceps, pronator terres, interosseous membrane, and finally the retinaculum. Finally, adding FOR in a regional approach to the shoulder area, it was possible to progressively isolate restriction deep in the components of the shoulder girdle and to begin to overcome the layers of overdevelopment and stress that had accumulated over years.

In this context, the stereognostic awareness that comes from the tactile feedback of applied oscillation is very much like sonar, where energy is sent into tissue and the response assessed for normal compliance. With rapidly repeated rhythmic input, assessing the quality, location, and angle of tissue compliance under controlled load, an image is created that either encourages one to persist and coax the tissue, or to modify one's efforts accordingly.

No manipulation is a matter of taking over the body's self-healing capacity. No medicine, even an alternative approach, is a method intended to control nature; hence the term "Facilitated" in this intended use of oscillatory force.

Another Way—Slow Rhythmic Oscillatory Release

Much of what I have described so far has relied on the idea of restoring neuromuscular balance through rhythmic entrainment. Another way to apply and conceptualize rhythmic manipulation is with a much slower cycle, and a different feel. This approach, in my thought, depends on the use of oscillatory force, converted into the energy of activation for another type of release.

The literature describes the elasticity of connective tissue and the distortion of fibrin through strain if the elastic limit is exceeded. In the process, bonds are released and reformed, accompanied by the ultimate release of energy. The process is termed hysteresis.

If on a microscopic and anatomical scale this results in the alteration of structure and function, balance can only be restored by the introduction of new energy of activation to catalyze the dissolution of the inappropriate dysfunctional bonds and the recreation of balance.

By applying slow rhythmic oscillation to the target tissue, one can introduce and catalyze or coax a release. Because the process is more deliberate, one must focus more precisely. However, in doing so, one can direct change to deeper or more delicate structures than in the previously described methods. Possibly this may also involve the resetting of postural neural pattern generators and reflexes through entrainment of their endogenous resonant frequency of depolarization.

Perhaps the difference in approach from conventional myofascial release can best be described in an example. If, in treating the right shoulder, it is determined that some of the restriction of motion comes from the glenohumeral joint, treatment can be directed there. Coupled diagnosis and treatment can be applied by grasping the joint anteriorly and posteriorly in the supine patient. If, in working with the right shoulder, the practitioner's left hand supports the proximal humerus from behind and lateral, the right hand gently but firmly closes in on the anterior or medial surface. The fingers can be spread to almost encircle the shoulder. Oscillatory motion would then be introduced by cyclically stretching the deep tissues, the capsular ligaments, in what would be a para-saggital plane, if the arm were at the patient's side. Working in a circular fashion, the upper arm would be brought forward, then superior, then posterior, then distal in smooth rhythmic circles in a 3- to 6-second frequency, depending on the proportions of practitioner and patient. By making the moves slower and more deliberate, slight variations in tension can be detected, very direct stretches can be integrated into the maneuver, and at the same time adjustments can be made to keep the treatment within the patient's comfort range, avoiding any potential guarding. Each aspect can increase effectiveness in a particular way.

The principles just described can be integrated into a variety of articular moves, including those for the hip joint, sacro-iliac joint, knee, or interphalangeal joints. Visualization of the local anatomy, expected native range of motion, and the target tissue improve the specificity and effectiveness of this work. Practice increases ease and the ability to more finely define treatment goals. The key is to use gently engaging, repetitive articular stretch.

Another means of using slow rhythm release is borrowed from the work of Elaine Wallace, DO, in her model termed *torque unwinding*. This material is not yet published other than in informal course notes.[1] There is much more to the model and it is well worth investigating. The portion that I find relevant here is her application of treatment force called *bouncing*.

In this model of myofascial-connective tissue work, the trunk and limbs are considered as divided functional regions visualized as blocks or cylindrical anatomical areas or spaces, defined largely by the diagonal patterns of muscle fibers that define regional motion and postural stability. The head-neck and thorax-abdomen would each form a functional block, with each extremity representing a cylinder. Often a painful, symptomatic area will be at one end of a diagonal fascial band in symmetric relationship around the center of mass of the block or cylinder to a tender point on the opposite side. To treat such a tender spot or symptom representing a point of fascial tightness, it is necessary to first identify both ends of this functional diagonal, representing each end of the involved fascial band, which is palpable as a point of increased tension. It is usually at a location 180 degrees in radial symmetry around the center mass of the functional block. Having identified the second spot, one can confirm the relationship by pushing and feeling the impulse transmitted through to the initial spot. One method of treating, then, is to push alternately on either end of this connective tissue couple, rhythmically, until a release occurs. In my view this is but another means of identifying target tissue.

An example of application would be a tenderness or sensitivity due to tension over a left first costovertebral joint. In this model the relevant anatomical block is the thorax and one would search out the corresponding tender spot on the right anterior lower thorax, perhaps near the costochondral joint of the tenth rib or tip of the eleventh or twelfth ribs.

A force applied diagonally in alternating directions between the points in a slow rhythmic cadence would be intended to release the fascial tension responsible for the symptom.

Summary

Although vibration or oscillation is not new to manipulative bodywork, FOR formalizes an approach to integrating this force into practice. It integrates seamlessly into combination or eclectic treatment. Most particularly it combines well with connective tissue release techniques, articular, muscle energy, and functional approaches. Additionally, my research into potential physiological mechanisms of effectiveness casts further light on potential mechanisms responsible for hypertonia contributing to the restriction of motion recognized by osteopathy as the root of much somatic dysfunction.

Reference

[1] Wallace, E., M. Goldman, and L. Boyajian. "Torque Unwinding," unpublished course notes from AAO Convocation workshop, 2004.

Chapter 12

Specific Regional Approaches

Lower-Extremity Leverage Techniques— Lumbar Spine, Pelvis, Hip, and Sacrum

In using rhythmic release for the sacrum, a simple rule of thumb applies. Regardless of one's diagnostic system (muscle energy, Chicago model, or other), the practitioner should apply steady force to the most posterior aspect of the sacrum with one hand, while adding rhythmic force with the other. How is this done? If treating a right posterior sacral base, while standing on the right side of the prone patient, grasp the right leg at the ankle, flex the knee, and add oscillations by rhythmic internal and external rotation of the thigh. If one finds this cumbersome, an alternative approach is to reach beneath the thigh, knee still bent, and cradle the entire limb. In this case, oscillations are lateral to medial but one can also rotate the thigh to find the position of laxity of the sacro-iliac joint. Either approach mobilizes the sacro-iliac joint, gapping it a bit in full internal rotation, and facilitates the sacrum returning anteriorly to a neutral position. The oscillation encourages it to float there rather than forcing the return.

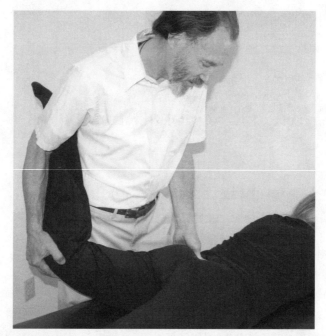

Figure 12-1. To reverse a sacrum held in extension, leg
leverage can be used to localize to the barrier. The bent knee
provides more control over the extremity. Oscillation is
generated by rhythmic motions of the practitioner's torso.

I have frequently found slow rhythmic release to be of value.
Often in a patient with psoas syndrome, a variety of spasm in a
major hip flexor, there is a group rotation of thoracic segment ten
(T10) down to the second lumbar segment (L2) toward the side of
most tension; in more extreme cases there may be an accentuated
rotation and sidebending, a non-physiological Fryette type two
dysfunction, toward the side of tension at T12 or L1. These are
painful. Conventional treatment might be to stretch and apply
muscle energy technique to the psoas, and then separately treat
the vertebral rotation. In FOR these can both be integrated into
the same set of movements, making the manipulation both more
effective and gentler.

When working with a right psoas in the prone patient, the practitioner stands on the patient's left side. The heel of the left hand, either pisiform or radial styloid process, is placed over the transverse process of the vertebral segment to be derotated (T12 or L1). The right hand reaches over and grasps the patient's right thigh just above the knee. Leaning one's body weight backwards, the right arm extends the hip and thigh until this extension reaches to and beyond the fulcrum created by the left hand. Refined localization, or resistive force, of the left hand while initiating a gentle rocking on this leverage, accentuating and releasing pressure on the psoas, may coax release and rotation simultaneously. This technique can be adapted to treatment of the seated patient for many segmental dysfunctions, but with gravity supplying the leg leverage.

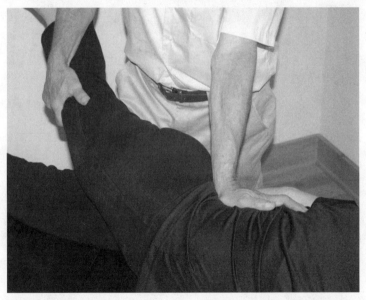

Figure 12-2. Treating right psoas tension, by creating a left rotation of T12 (or L1) with the activating hand over the left transverse process. Use the leg to stretch the psoas, while gently rocking.

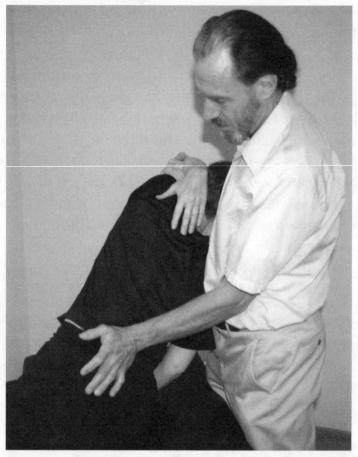

Figure 12-3. A similar strategy may be applied with the patient seated, when convenient. Gravity provides lower-extremity resistance against torso torsion.

All this is done within the comfort limitations of the patient. In the acute spasm there typically may be reactive guarding, in which case an indirect technique such as counterstrain may be more effective.

In further applying this derotation maneuver, the lower extremity may be used rhythmically to apply diagnostic and general treatment pressure up and down the spinal column in the prone position, as in mobilizing the spine, described at the beginning of Chapter 10. Accentuation of the pressure may establish what John Wernham calls "specific treatment within the context of general treatment."[1] If less force is required, leverage can be applied using the right hand to grasp the contralateral ileum. A further variation used in seated or prone position is the use of the thumb as a fulcrum, illustrated again here (see detail in Figure 12-5). Such a pattern allows for more focal application of force, and a more precise localization over a transverse process leading to an overall more delicate treatment. In so doing, we are applying the dynamic rhythmic equivalent of Wernham's "dog" technique.

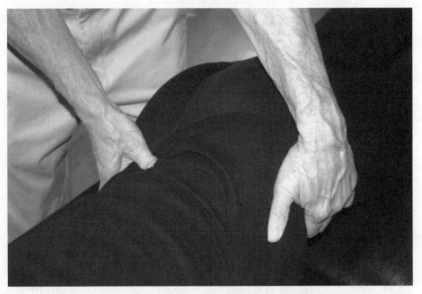

Figure 12-4. Lumbar treatment can be localized by grasping as shown, leaning body weight to develop myofascial localization, with activating force developed then by rhythmic rocking of the practitioner's body.

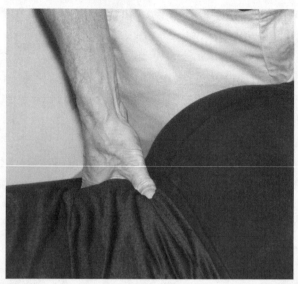

Figure 12-5. The thumb can be used as a firm point of contact to localize vibratory force.

Putting many of these elements illustrated thus far, we can find an effective alternative means of treating and sidebending L5. In treating a dysfunctional L5 segment, both common and painful and often presenting as sciatica, a similar combination of strategies can be applied. The lower extremity again is used for leverage and thumb pressure is applied as follows. Presuming a left rotated L5, one would stand on the right side of the prone patient and place one's left thumb firmly over the most posterior, the left, transverse process, thus rotating the vertebra to the right. Presuming Fryette's biomechanics, this would be coupled to a left sidebending. To right sidebend the target segment, one would lift and place the right then left lower extremity to the right sidebent position, probably with feet and legs off the table. Firm pressure with the practitioner's body weight behind it, accompanied by assurance and instruction for the patient not to "help you," adds to the success of this treatment. Should the patient introduce voluntary motion to assist in repositioning, the effectiveness of connective tissue stretch is compromised.

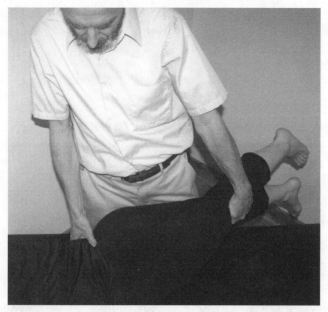

Figure 12-6. L5, representing a transition zone between functional anatomical regions, often becomes restricted. An effective strategy applies leg leverage to derotate and for sidebending against the restricted barrier, with oscillatory force before isometric contraction.

With the patient placed in this intended right rotation and sidebending, the further introduction of force proceeds with deep pressure, with slight rhythmic variation, and respiratory cooperation. (Pressure is accentuated during the relaxation of exhalation phase of respiration.) If respiratory cooperation is to be optimized, ask the patient to take a deep breath, coax him or her to go deeper, and then ask the patient to cough the breath out all at one time. The more punctual the expulsion of breath, the more extreme the exhalation, the more effective is the force of respiratory cooperation.

Added activating force may be applied through steady or rhythmic leverage of the lower extremity by shifting the practitioner's body weight. Muscle energy may be added by telling the patient to push the leg forward as in the effort to take a step. If necessary, a short thrust can also be applied. All compatible techniques may be applied sequentially in an eclectic fashion.

Supine Lower-Extremity Applications

In articular or myofascial direct release, we can use oscillation to enhance release in most planes in the hip, knee, or fibular region, whether the target is clearly defined or not. We have only to visualize the tissue and adjust traction until we feel the desired localization. Whenever the direct barrier is engaged, oscillatory force can expedite advancement of the barrier alone, or in combination with sequential direct stretch, or isometric contraction followed by release (muscle energy technique). The oscillatory release works well to further localize the barrier and refine muscle energy technique.

If one is accustomed to subtle work, including indirect myofascial release, balanced ligamentous tension, or fluidic approaches, gentle oscillatory vibration in the mid-zone between tensions (for example, between internal and external rotation of the knee) seems to expedite release. The method is especially beneficial in the context of acute strain or trauma since it is so gentle and avoids involuntary antalgic guarding of inflamed tissues. This strategy would apply also to ankle sprain, a common injury pattern. The intended effect is to offer the connective tissue matrix, including the colloidal ground substance, an opportunity to reorganize and redistribute inherent forces. Issues related to energetics, hysteresis, and balancing tensions are all potentially relevant here. The technique may also be applied to acute or chronically inflamed knees or digits.

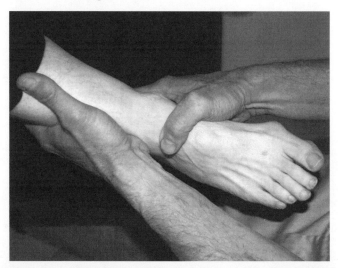

Figure 12-7. Oscillation can be used in the context of indirect myofascial release to diffuse the residual tension after acute injury, such as ankle sprain.

Seated Shoulder and Upper-Extremity Leverage Techniques

The introductory techniques described above for lumbar spine address the trunk, but in the prone position; the spine is already placed in some degree of extension. If a thoracic segment is restricted and held in a relative extension position, this is not an optimally effective position from which to induce segmental flexion. It may be possible to restore motion by focusing attention on the rotational component and introducing motion through the transverse process. However, if further flexion is required, a seated treatment position may be preferred. In this position, the shoulders or upper extremity can be used to first put the torso in tension to localize, then introduce the appropriate articular oscillatory force.

In treating a typical thoracic vertebra in the T4–T8 range that is extended, the following strategies may be used to introduce oscillatory force. The practitioner asks the patient to sit with arms crossed on the chest and approaches the patient from behind, from the side to which rotation and sidebending are to be introduced. Reaching across the spine, place the heel of the hand or the thumb as a fulcrum on the posterior transverse process of the appropriate segment. If treating a T5 rotated left, sidebent left and extended, approach from the right and place the left thumb or heel of the hand over the left transverse process. Place the right arm around in front of the patient over the patient's right shoulder, wrapping the arm across the upper chest, and placing the practitioner's right hand on the patient's left shoulder. The practitioner's upper arm or axilla should rest on the patient's right shoulder. To create the potential space for articular release, first one adds compression through the arm or axilla on the patient's right shoulder, proceeding to add sidebending and slight rotation to the right. Next, localization to the restrictive barrier is accomplished by first smoothly sidebending *left* by pressing down on the left shoulder while shifting the patient's center of gravity right, which causes the patient's hips to shift right to create a counter force for the sidebending. Then rotation is completed by rotating the right shoulder anterior. This is accomplished by the practitioner rotating his or her right shoulder anterior. Flexion is added by the practitioner leaning forward, now almost over the patient.

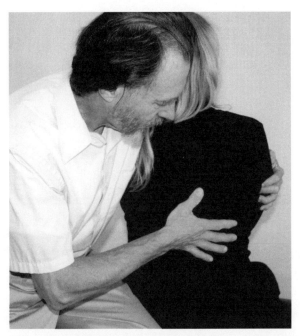

Figure 12-8. Oscillation can be integrated into any seated positional treatment, such as functional release, thrust, articular, or muscle energy techniques.

This description seems counterintuitive since we are sidebending and rotating the shoulders in the direction of the restriction. But our intent is to oppose the motion of shoulders and the dysfunctional segment by the direction of the thumb.

Once this motion pattern is understood, it is clear that one cycle represents an attempt at articular release. In classical articular technique, this motion would be repeated for several discrete cycles. In oscillatory release, this pattern could be smoothly repeated, beginning with gentle excursions, then with progressing to extent of motion in each plane, depending on the degree of resistance appreciated. Once rhythmic motion is established, the fulcrum hand can be moved up or down the thoracic cage and spine to eliminate any residual, or newly discovered, resistance in ribs or other spinal segments. The pattern of dynamic motion refines diagnosis, focuses treatment, and imparts a feeling of relaxation to the patient.

By now, hopefully, the reader can see a pattern of setting up for muscle energy treatment and this is often the derivation of this localization. However, once the restrictive barrier is approached the application of force in FOR is different, but may be used before or after the application of muscle energy technique. If we rhythmically rotate the patient's torso through this direct approach to the restricted barrier, then back to its lesioned position, we have articular technique. If we pause at the barrier position, and add leverage through the right shoulder in the rotation, or sidebending component, we can have a uniquely FOR approach, introducing a rhythmic springing-type oscillatory force.

If we were treating a segment that was restricted in going into extension, the rotation and sidebending components would be similar in setup but the trunk would be extended around the fulcrum hand, using the shoulders for leverage. To apply oscillatory force, thumb pressure would be maintained and further extension would be induced by repetitively rocking the torso using the shoulder contact. This method is effective for reducing restriction in an elevated, posteriorly subluxed or inhalation rib by moving the thumb just lateral to the transverse process.

If one is uncomfortable with this torso-to-torso technique, similar leverages may be introduced using the patient's bent arm as leverage. This can be done in one of two ways. In traditional muscle energy work, this can be done by having the patient bend the left elbow and place the hand behind the neck. This is the arm on the side opposite that to which sidebending and rotation are to be introduced. The patient's other (right) hand grasps the left elbow. The practitioner then reaches across in front of the patient, going under the right arm and placing his or her right hand over the left bicep of the bent arm or grasping the flexed elbow in the palm.

I prefer the following method because it develops more mechanical advantage. The patient bends the left elbow, with hand behind neck as before; however, the shoulder is flexed to bring the elbow up to being level with the top of the head. This provides a lever for more effective sidebending coupled to the rotation (see Figure 12-9). With either contact, the torso can be easily sidebent, rotated, flexed, or extended in the desired direction. Oscillator force would be introduced by a gentle springing motion against the restrictive barrier through this leverage.

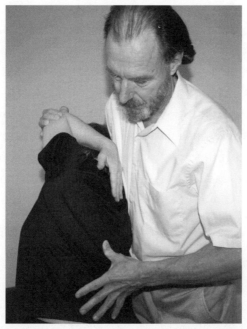

Figure 12-9. For those preferring a more direct approach to the dysfunctional barrier, mechanical advantage can be increased, but gently, adding the bent arm for additional leverage. Oscillations allow the force to be transmitted gently but effectively.

The advantage of the bent-arm technique is the development of power from a longer lever arm to overcome the articular restriction. However, I prefer the tighter technique described first, since it allows more immediate feedback and more delicate localization, which is a key feature to the effectiveness of slow-rhythm FOR.

Supine Upper-Extremity Leverage Techniques

Basic supine upper-extremity techniques have been introduced in the basic exercises in Chapter 10. As mentioned then, because of the degrees of freedom of motion of the upper extremity, it is difficult to localize force specifically beyond the scapulothoracic and sternoclavicular articulations. However, with torsion and thoughtful, precise localization, the arm can be used to leverage and rhythmically treat the thoracic spine and rib cage.

One example is articular treatment of the first rib, which, because of its intimate association with the clavicle and scapula, is affected by arm motion, especially abduction. However, many potential dysfunctions may exist in the shoulder complex and in the more distal extremity. Treatment of most will involve regional or broad fascial application of force because of the nature and distribution of fascia along the planes of the trapezius, latissimus, and pectoralis muscles.

With care, the abducted and externally rotated arm may be used, with practitioner's hand or table as a fulcrum under the humeral head, to promote articular movement of the costovertebral joints. When necessary, the fingers of the posterior hand may direct force to the rib heads and adjacent tissues. This combined technique can be useful in cases of upper-extremity repetitive strain syndrome, thoracic outlet syndrome, or acute or chronic bronchitis. Tension in the pectoral musculature, and related regional restriction of motion, is the target of treatment here.

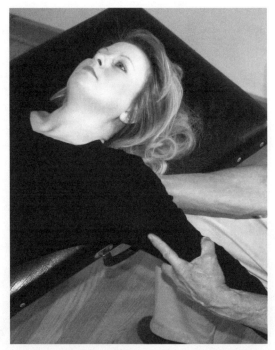

Figure 12-10. Tension in the pectoralis minor muscle, often associated with brachial plexus compression syndromes, can be approached in such a manner as illustrated.

To refine the technique, stand beside the supine patient, on the side to be treated, facing the patient's feet. Abduct the patient's arm, adding spiral fascial traction (external for upper ribs, internal for lower ribs) to tighten the fascia of the shoulder and upper arm. Stabilize and control movement of this arm with your right arm. The heel of the left hand cushions and diffuses strain to the glenohumeral joint, while the fingertips probe to localize motion to the rib heads or costovertebral joints. Adjustments or accommodations will need to be made according to the proportions and constitution of patient and practitioner. Once positioned, an oscillatory rocking, allowing the patient's arm to drop gently toward the floor while the practitioner uses the left thenar-hypothenar eminence as a fulcrum, enables the fingertips to rhythmically probe and articulate the rib heads and adjacent tissue. The practitioner's two hands work in harmonic, rhythmic, reciprocal motion to relax and loosen tissue. The dialogue with the patient is aimed at coaxing, not forcing, change.

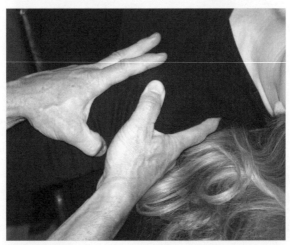

Figure 12-11. In complex regions such as the shoulder, two hands working as a team can add precision in treatment. Oscillations add a further dimension of force to the precise myofascial stretch and kneading.

Supine Cervical Technique

Supine application to the cervical region mirrors that described for supine thoracic work, with regional accommodations to the nature of the functional anatomy. Because of the complexity of the region, I describe technique here only for the typical cervical vertebra C2–C6. Those with an interest in refined application can extrapolate from a more complete osteopathic treatment of the region as described elsewhere.[2]

Whether in flexion or extension, we treat by approaching the barrier. However, because of the extreme flexibility and coupled motion in sidebending and rotation of cervical vertebrae, I rely on treating with localization toward the restriction of motion in one of these two classic planes of motion, with the other taking the opposite direction for each setup. In other words, for a vertebral segment that is restricted in flexion, sidebending right, rotation right, treatment would be directed toward the flexion restriction and either the right rotational or sidebending restriction. The other element would be addressed differently. In setting up for direct technique, the remaining parameter (sidebending or rotation) would be taken in the opposite direction. In fact, all the regional segments would be taken in the opposite direction from the restricted segmental barrier in order to further localize the potential effect of the activating force at the intended segment. This is necessary because of the extreme flexibility or freedom of motion of the cervical spine.

Having clarified these practice conventions, in treating C4, which is at ease in flexion, sidebending right, rotation left (restricted sidebending left, rotation right), the direct treatment might involve regional sidebending right, extension against resistance, then inducing left rotation of C4. This would be accomplished by sitting at the head of the patient, using the side of the left index metacarpal or phalangeal joint to create a fulcrum at the segment below.

The activating oscillatory force could be applied in two ways. Either the right hand of the practitioner could support the patient's head and create very gentle left rotational spring in opposition to the fulcrum stabilization of the opposing hand. Or, with the hands in the same positions, the right hand could guide the head away from the barrier (to the right) then re-approach the barrier in a rhythmic articular manner. Often this approach would be used in combination with articular, myofascial or muscle energy treatment in a smooth blend.

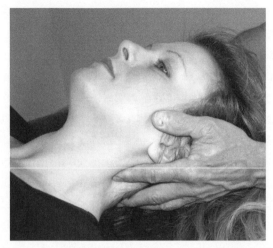

Figure 12-12. Cervical manipulation can be delicate in the case of the osteoarthritic patient. Vibratory force allows the treatment to proceed within the comfort range of the patient but quickly, precisely, and effectively.

Cranial Flutter Techniques

By following the rationale and implementation of technique thus far, the reader can see that oscillatory release integrates with other methods in a wide variety of clinical situations. I do not presume to appreciate all the permutations of conditions. There are even applications in the context of cranial work. The following are several examples.

Focal oscillatory inhibition has been described above. In this situation, a small tissue target is contacted by the index finger tip and oscillation applied by developing the standing wave in the practitioner's arm. Rhythmically moving the flexed elbow toward and away from one's body, the practitioner develops a standing sinusoidal wave in his or her own arm. This rhythmic momentum can then be imparted through the contacting finger tip to the patient's body as needed in discrete, small areas.

It may additionally be applied to the tightened muscles of the sub-occipital triangle affecting the gliding of the occipital condyles; similarly, it can be directed toward the insertion of the splenius capitis or sternocleidomastoid muscles in torticollis.

Additionally, in cases of temporomandibular joint dysfunction, this force may be used to loosen the ligaments of the tighter, more restricted mastoid condylar joint.

In a more general treatment mode, oscillation can be imparted in any conventional cranial contact or "hold" by reciprocally fluttering the hands in opposite directions. Applying this strategy, I will assess membranous or osseous restriction and very gently quiver my hands at about 300 cycles per minute for 5 or 6 seconds to coax the intended motion. Such a strategy implies the capacity of the practitioner to define normal motion and restriction in the cranial field.

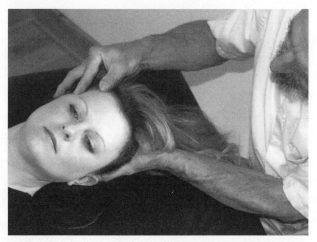

Figure 12-13. Within one's confidence level, gentle vibratory force can enhance other forces in application in the cranial area.

This approach can be applied not only in a subtle biomechanical framework. It can be applied if one works with restrictions in the membranes or fluidic milieu of the patient. Specificity of visualization is what is important.

It is not presumed that this applies only to adult patients. If done gently, this can be included in the treatment of infants. Remember that babies enjoy being rocked. Rhythmic motion is natural to them and soothing. Singing to their children has been a natural transcultural practice for mothers forever—an intimate application of interpersonal vibration. If you have natural pitch, do not hesitate to sing or hum as you work.

Again, in this region, the reader is reminded to pay attention to practicing within the scope of one's license, training, and area of expertise. Though apparently gentle and benign, application of nonphysiological force in critical areas can, in some cases, have significant and not always desirable impact. Proceed ethically and respectfully.

Yet Another, Subtle Mode of FOR

As discussed, FOR may well be considered an extension of connective tissue manipulation or myofascial release, applying the principle of longitudinal stretch to tight tissues but in *small bites* rather than long linear stretch. A variety of osteopathic approaches have evolved that focus predominantly on functional considerations and transfer the principles of palpation and motion testing in a very subtle mode or sphere of focus. Cranial, functional methods, visceral manipulation, somato-emotional release, and subtle mode connective tissue release all pay attention to a level of concentration and refinement that is practical if cultivated but appears to be delusional behavior to those who have not acquired the interest or skill. It is recognized that there is a legitimate variety of gifts, talents, and ways of knowing. In this context we have tried to develop in the background for FOR

a conceptual bridge between subtle methods and a newer generation of accepted neurophysiology.

But for those so inclined, FOR implemented on a subtle scale
is a useful tool for the appropriate patient. An application that
immediately comes to mind is the elderly patient with neck
pain and headache, who has a moderate degree of osteoarthritic
change. This is the patient in whom we should be reticent to do
high-velocity low-amplitude thrust despite our earnest desire to
help. Yet a direct technique, in this difficult and uncomfortable
patient, assures him or her of our recognition of the problem, our
intention to help, and our competency. In a non-FOR context, safe
methods would be traction followed by gentle ligamentous stretch
plus articulation. Muscle energy technique, controlled for comfort
of the patient, would be a further conservative approach.

FOR can be integrated early in the process. Working with the
patient in a seated position, where he or she has come to rest,
paraspinous palpation can demonstrate segmental positional
asymmetry, if present. If one introduces simultaneous gentle
oscillatory counter-rotations from a hand placed over the head
and one spanning the transverse articular pillars at each successive segment, restriction of motion can be detected. To treat in
this gentle mode, one can oscillate in neutral or can also accentuate the articular aspect of the treatment by adding sidebending
directly to the barrier while continuing the vibrations. At any
time the application of force in many other styles may complement the oscillation.

In the description of treating the ankle, above, reference was
made to treating in the style of indirect myofascial release. How
does one make this indirect technique work? The answer lies in cul-
tivating an educated sense of tissue ease. The functional-methods
approach of Johnston pays attention to tissue texture quality, ease
versus bind, at the very beginning of introduced motion.

Indirect connective tissue release depends on an ability to sense such ease in successive dimensions progressively and to follow this shifting balance point to a new resting state. In doing such there is the assumption that by adding corrective afferent input below the threshold of nociception, sympathetic hyper-arousal, and guarding, the nervous system recognizes its state of native rest. By adding subtle FOR, the effect may be amplified, gently increasing the degree of comfort and relaxation in an area previously only noticeable by stress and pain. Another possible mechanism is the entrainment of a resonant state of phase coherence among the neurons associated with a previously induced muscle spasm or persistent contracted state.

Diagnosis or assessment in this subtle field is enhanced by the development of stereognosis, or a sense of tactile spatial discrimination. Like using tactile sonar, in application in a case of thoracic outlet syndrome, one would start gently as in general listening, bounce out a wave with rhythmic motions through the shoulder musculature, looking for response, and then follow the tightness and engage it with progressive specificity until as much as possible of the pathologic barrier is erased and natural motion restored.

The Horizon

This book and the proposition of application of oscillatory force under the name Facilitated Oscillatory Release is not meant to be purely imitative, nor is it intended to be viewed as revelatory or conclusive. Rather, it is intended to widen the scope of application of intentional force to the body, compatible with the body's internal rhythmic, regulatory processes.

In trying to transform medical practice by attending to the physical relationships of the body, and admonishing practitioners to find the unnatural associated with disease and return it to the natural state, Andrew Still did not intend to apply a different but confined perimeter to treatment options. He intended to be comprehensive in his approach to facilitating natural function.

Since early osteopathic time, and in other contexts, oscillation and vibration have been intuitively applied to promote health. They have been a part of other bodywork approaches. Reaching for understanding and explanations, practitioners and scientists have found themselves wandering in many directions, often esoteric and idiosyncratic in their interests and expression. The mainstream health care culture would like to express itself in the empirical, bioscientific paradigm. And so, in many circles, energetics, vibration, and oscillation presented in esoteric language have become awkward, uncomfortable baggage to some, but natural to many, representing the application of rhythmic, harmonic force to restore health.

This book, and the FOR method, are intended to help add further credibility to this quest to further understand the nature of the human person as a harmonic structure and the search for further scientific understanding. It is also intended to lend support to all those who have persisted in appreciating the naturalness of rhythmic, harmonic processes in understanding disease and promoting health.

I thank the reader for persisting to this point and look forward to collegial development of a community of understanding in this exciting area of health care research and practice.

References

[1] Wernham, J., and C. Campbell. *The Osteopathic Technique and Philosophy of John Wernham,* video (Maidstone, England: Institute of Classical Osteopathy, 1996).

[2] Essig-Beatty, D. *Pocket Manual of OMT* (Lewisburg: West Virginia School of Osteopathic Medicine, 2004), 248.

Appendix A

Osteopathic Approach
to Health Care in Context

Early Development

After losing his first wife and several of his children to what he ascribed to be the inadequacies of current health care, Andrew Still began a course of further personal study to improve his medical practice. Much of this study, during the 1860s, involved a review of anatomy and physiology from the point of view of observation of nature. He derived conclusions regarding causation and treatment that differed significantly from the conventional views of his day.

Among these were the appreciation of what would in our day be described as the importance of competence of the cardiovascular system, proper function of neural transmitters and neural reflexes, the role of hemoglobin in red blood cells, and the role of the immune system in fighting disease. Much of the proper function of these systems would be described as dependent on local and regional anatomical integrity of both structure and function. Distortions of the musculoskeletal and other systems and tissues supporting function resulted in suboptimal function. Improper function of the musculoskeletal system, and therefore the other systems and total health, could be improved by manual adjustments. "Find the unnatural and return it to the natural" was the guide to treatment.

As Still opened a school to teach his methods in 1892, his teaching evolved in dialogue with his students. Many of his students began to write their own textbooks on the subject of osteopathy, variously emphasizing different aspects of Still's thought, but none attained the comprehensive approach inherent in Dr. Still's work.

While stressing the anatomy, Still would also reflect that the patient was a composite of body, mind, and spirit and could not be dealt with by attending to just one aspect. Although many of his thoughts ring true with the complementary and alternative medicine of our day, reading Still is difficult, partly because of his personal writing style, the vernacular of his day, and the state of the art of medicine and then-current pattern of defining issues.

Despite the breadth of his thought, Still was a practical man. He made diverse speculations about the nature of man, of life, and medical practice. However, in describing and defending his school and methods, he presented a reductionistic approach to osteopathy to the public, emphasizing treatment by manual manipulation. Indeed, this was a distinguishing characteristic of the approach. This tactic eventually resulted in the recognition of osteopathy as a legitimate approach to medicine and the licensing of practitioners in all the states of the U.S. The struggle proceeded with the support of a broadening patient base, including those among the various legislatures, despite strong resistance from the organized medical community. The famous Samuel Clemens, AKA Mark Twain, made an eloquent defense for osteopathy before the New York state legislature.

With the legal acceptance of osteopathy came the issue of patient protection and quality standards in education. As a result of the Flexner Report and political support for the scientific basis for medicine, there came to be significant similarity between the osteopathic and allopathic medical curriculum except for the different emphasis on the study of functional anatomy. Eventually, surgery was added to osteopathic practice when necessary. Osteopathy proper sometimes described manipulation as "bloodless surgery." Pharmacology was crude and rejected by Still and his followers.

During this period of early solidification of osteopathy in the American political and social context, John Martin Littlejohn formally introduced osteopathy to the British Isles. A Scotsman, Littlejohn and his brothers had initially been patients, then students, then faculty, at Still's American School of Osteopathy. They differed from Still in regard to physiological concepts and political tactics, but not in spirit of the importance of anatomy or manual intervention. However, their divisions helped define the two main developmental tracks in osteopathy and led to the varied expression of osteopathic activity that we see today internationally—the physician and the non-physician osteopathic practitioner.

As a result of Still's initial effort in the ASO's home state of Missouri, he was granted recognition and the privilege to grant MD degrees. Feeling this would mute the distinctiveness of osteopathic practice, Still chose to call his graduates *"Diplomats* of Osteopathy"—DOs. Osteopaths internationally retain this designation after osteopathic training. In the U.S., the initials were later redesignated to represent the degree of *Doctor* of Osteopathy and eventually diplomas have come to bear the title Doctor of Osteopathic Medicine.

Through long struggle against medical resistance, DOs in the U.S. gained first the right to participate as medical officers in medical military service in the mid-1960s. This was followed by state-by-state acceptance of the osteopathic national educational competency exam and the community-by-community granting of medical privileges in allopathic hospitals. With the restructuring of the health care business in the 1990s and the consolidation of multiple hospitals under corporate umbrellas, many osteopathic hospitals lost their independent governance.

Since osteopathic education had kept pace with the standard of medical education and care, osteopathic physicians found increased ease in gaining specialty and general medical attending privileges in mixed-staff hospitals. With this development, physicians in residency training from osteopathic schools demonstrated the distinctiveness of osteopathic medicine practice to a wider audience of patients and physicians.

Osteopathic Practice Today

So how might an osteopathic medical approach differ from the care rendered by the majority medical profession? I will state at the beginning of this section that there is a broad spectrum of interest among osteopathic graduates on this issue. Many would prefer being perceived as totally equivalent to their medical colleagues. Others, admittedly a minority, embrace a distinctively different approach to care. Most are somewhere in between. But let us use the example of a patient presenting to the family physician with a headache.

The first concern in either camp would be to determine if the headache represents a critical or acutely emergent condition. Vital signs, including blood pressure, connected with the patient's complaint and the relevant history developed through a dialogue would guide this process. Especially for a headache, the history of frequency, duration, and location of pain can often describe the type of headache. Screening and confirmatory diagnostic testing, including imaging studies, might be ordered if deemed appropriate. An evaluation of the head, including carotid artery sounds, along with inspection of eyes, ears, nose, and throat, besides the blood pressure measurement, would be basic. Some simple tests of neural function would be part of the workup.

The osteopathic physician would be equipped, if he or she chose, to go more thoroughly into the physical examination. Palpation, or discriminative touch, would be used to identify muscle tension in the neck and upper back that might be referring, or creating tension, in the scalp or head. Restriction of mobility in the otherwise flexible spine of the neck might also give similar pain patterns. Symmetry of position and subtle movement of the cranial bones may aid some specially trained osteopaths in refining the diagnosis.

Special attention would be paid, in the osteopathic context, to the body's memory of old trauma. The fascial or connective tissue of the body is treated as if it were a reservoir for strain resulting from trauma sometimes much earlier in life. The emotional memory of an unpleasant or traumatic event might also be considered in some cases.

A common headache pattern derives from anxiety, perceived stress, and the resultant muscle tension. Besides reducing this tension by physical means (manipulation) or by pharmaceutical means, the osteopath would tend to consider the social context and personal behavior of the patient in creating, and perhaps resolving, the pattern of tension associated with the headache.

One might say, well, this is only good and compassionate medical care. However, osteopathy tries to maintain a culture of sensitivity, attentive to scientific knowledge of the integration of body systems, compatible with the growing awareness of complementary and alternative care.

In his early writing, Dr. Still suggested addressing the patient as a complex whole:

First there is the physical body, then the spiritual body, and the body of mind.

As noted earlier in the book, osteopathy today formulates the principles derived from Still, as follows:

1. The human being is a dynamic unit of function.
2. The body possesses self-regulatory mechanisms that are self-healing in nature.
3. Structure and function are interrelated at all levels.
4. Rational treatment is based on these principles.

Although there is no proprietary restriction on the use of these principles, they are reiterated in the course of osteopathic education. Combined with the importance of personal touch and relationship that develops around this aspect of the encounter, the principles provide a platform for a distinctive approach to health care.

Osteopathic manipulation has remained one of the distinctive features of the osteopathic approach. From the start, osteopathy emphasized the optimization of function through the correction of structural problems. Early on, these problematic areas in the body were referred to as the "osteopathic lesion." Attempts were made to define, in a physiological sense, what they represented. The role of tissue swelling or edema, of muscle tension, of fixations or subluxations of joints, and neural reflexes were all explored. In the 1960s a team of experts, attempting to communicate with insurance companies over the issue of reimbursement, arrived at a definition for the osteopathic lesion, modernized in the terminology of somatic dysfunction.[1]

Since there have existed differences of opinion in the physiological research community, as well as in the practitioner community over the basis for somatic dysfunction, the definition attempted to be comprehensive, underscoring the osteopathic principle of the body as a functional unity. Over time, various approaches or schools of osteopathic technique developed. Each came from the clinical experience of one or several practitioners in relation to their success in treatment. Hypothetical models for the success of the various techniques developed over time, modified by progressive scientific learning and discovery.

A list of the various major technical approaches would include:

Myofascial/connective tissue release
Strain counterstrain
Muscle energy
Functional methods
Cranial osteopathy
High-velocity, low-amplitude thrust techniques

An individual practitioner might practice using only one preferred technique, or several. Often a practitioner with the desire for further learning incorporates principles from several technical models in an eclectic, unique way as an artist combines colors, a musician combines notes, to create the desired effect. In this way, treatment is customized to meet the needs of the individual patient.

Interdisciplinary Cooperation

Compatibility, reciprocal referrals, and cooperation between bodyworkers and other health care providers vary with geographic and social context. Because osteopathy in the U.S. is embedded in medical practice, cooperation between MDs and DOs is complex. In the aspect of general and specialty practice, both accept each other as peers. Although in the past, there was general skepticism among many MDs about the relevance or validity of osteopathic manipulation, this attitude seems to be changing. Collegial relationships in mixed-staff hospitals, with the inclusion of students in residency training in such settings, has tended to increase mutual understanding. Manual diagnosis and treatment increasingly are being correctly demonstrated, understood, and valued.

The relationship between physical therapists and osteopathic physicians has been increasingly cordial and complementary. Physical therapists have progressively received more referrals from osteopathic, as well as allopathic, physicians. A number of defined osteopathic technical approaches have been adopted by physical therapists and other bodyworkers. Other techniques have been independently derived but share the same physiological concepts and similar applications. These have included myofascial release, counterstrain, muscle energy technique, and cranial work.

In the U.S., competition for business, as well as an early historic rivalry, have been more present between osteopaths and chiropractic practitioners. There is some overlap in technique in certain areas but also significant differences, both in diagnostic modalities and monitoring changes during and after treatment. Cooperation between local individual practitioners is not uncommon.

Outside the U.S., these relationships are somewhat different. To begin, there is no medically oriented pre-doctoral training. A previous education and practice in physiotherapy or another line of bodywork may qualify a person for training as an osteopath. The recommendation for such international programs is for a minimum of four years of part-time study, often amounting to 2,000 hours of supervised instruction or clinical practice. This avenue follows the Littlejohn model of practice. Progressively more countries are accepting and regulating this model where it exists.

The second avenue of osteopathic practice consists of physicians, usually with an orientation to sports medicine, physical medicine, or orthopedics, who seek out additional osteopathic training. Programs usually amount to 400 to 700 hours of instruction, mostly in technique.

A third group of DOs practicing overseas are American graduates who have sought to practice in another country.

Reference

[1] Ward, Robert, ed. *Foundations for Osteopathic Medicine,* 2nd ed. (Philadelphia: Lippincott Williams and Wilkins, 2003), 1227–1253.

Index

About the Author

Currently a resident of Lewisburg, West Virginia, Zachary Comeaux is an associate professor and practicing physician at the West Virginia School of Osteopathic Medicine.

The topics of Facilitated Oscillatory Release presented in this book and Bioenergetically Integrated Osteopathic Medicine have been the subject of workshops and addresses in Europe, South America, and Asia.

Born in the Philadelphia suburbs, Comeaux received a broad education due to diversity of interests. Before receiving a bachelor's degree in philosophy, he had pursued studies in psychology, mechanical engineering, and languages, besides developing a strong avocational interest in natural science. Comeaux received a degree of Doctor of Osteopathic Medicine after graduate-level studies in theology and clinical psychology and working in various social work venues. Influences from many of these disciplines find expression in his expanded approach to bodywork. Often, the phrases "energy medicine" or "alternative medicine" reflect a similar effort to reach for a higher level of understanding than normative practice.

Dr. Comeaux is certified in Family Medicine from the American Osteopathic Board of Family Practice and holds a certificate of special proficiency from the American Osteopathic Board of Neuromuscular Medicine. He is a member of the American Osteopathic Association (AOA) and American Academy of Osteopathy (AAO). He holds an earned Fellowship of the AAO. He is also a founding member of the Executive Committee of the World Osteopathic Health Organization.

He has been a thesis juror for the College d'Études d'Osteo-pathie, Canada, the Deutsche Osteopathishe Kolleg, Germany, and the Escola Brasileira de Osteopatia, Brazil. Comeaux has authored *Robert Fulford, DO, and the Philosopher Physician* and contributed to *Doctor Fulford's Touch of Life;* he is a contributing author to *A Pocket Manual of OMT: Osteopathic Manipulative Treatment for Physicians* (Essig-Beatty), *Cranial Manipulation Theory and Practice,* 2nd ed. (Chaitow), and *Somatic Dysfunction in Osteopathic Family Medicine* (Nelson). Additionally, he is a reviewer for the *Journal of Body Work and Movement Therapies* and the *Journal of the American Osteopathic Association.* A list of other journal articles and other information is available at zacharycomeaux.com.

Besides love for his work, Comeaux enjoys gardening, wood-carving, canoeing, and hiking in the forest. He shares these interests with his wife, Linda.